New Workout

Human Resistance Training

Dynamic Strength Training Without Equipment

John Laurie & Bum Lee

Cycle Publishing / Van der Plas Publications, San Francisco

copyright © 2004, John Laurie and Bum Lee

Printed in the USA
First edition, paperback original, 2004

Publisher's information:
Cycle Publishing / Van der Plas Publications
1282 7th Avenue
San Francisco, CA 94122
USA
http://www.cyclepublishing.com
E-mail: pubrel@cyclepublishing.com

Distributed or represented to the book trade by:
USA: Midpoint Trade Books, Kansas City, KS
UK: Chris Lloyd Sales and Marketing Services/Orca Book Services, Poole, Dorset
Australia: Tower Books, Frenchs Forest, NSW

Cover design:
Kent Lytle, Lytle Design, Alameda, CA
Cover photographs by Belda Photography, Emeryville, CA

Text photographs by John Laurie

Publisher's Cataloging in Publication Data
John Laurie and Lee, Bum. New Workout: Human Resistance Training. Dynamic Strength Training without Equipment.
I. Title: Dynamic Strength Training without Equipments.
II. Authorship: Lee, Bum, coauthor.
Bibliography, 168 p. 23 cm. Includes index.
ISBN 1-892495-44-9, trade paperback.
1. Health and Fitness, manuals and handbooks
2. Physical Exercise, manuals and handbooks
Library of Congress Control Number 2003115532

Acknowledgements

First and foremost, I would like to extend a special thank you to Don Williams. When I was just beginning in the fitness industry, Don was kind enough to take me under his wing. I am especially grateful for this considering the nature of the fitness profession, in which many trainers feel threatened by and show animosity toward others. Don never hesitated to show me what he knew, from various strength-training techniques to lessons on physiology and everything in between. One of the most knowledgeable trainers I have ever met, Don is rarely seen without strength-training literature, continually dissecting it in an attempt to glean even a little more knowledge and understanding of our complex field. Don has been a mentor, business partner, and I'm glad to say a friend. He has helped to invent or perfect a number of exercises within the pages of this book, and can truly be considered one of the founding fathers of modern Human Resistance Training. I would also like to thank my parents, David and Sandra Laurie, without whom, this book would not have been possible. Additionally, I would like to extend my gratitude to Steve Orris, an assistant strength coach at the University of Florida, who has helped me work through the logistics of applying Human Resistance Training to group settings and for sport specific purposes.

John Laurie

I would like to thank my parents, Seung and Jung Lee for their support. They exposed me to a wide range of sports and physical activity, which later developed into a love for fitness and exercise. I would also like to thank Richard Graham for taking me under his wing when I was just a teenager, and showing me the door to fitness. From there, I gained an understanding for the complexity of our industry. He showed me the literature of Joe Wieder, Author Jones, and Mike Mentzer. I would also like to thank Mike Merced, Sean Fazende, Jason Vaughn, and Joy Boudreaux, who have gone through many rigorous training days with me, during the experiment and exploration of my fitness evolution. Finally, I would like to thank professors Barbara Warren PhD, Gary Granata PhD, Jasper Loftin PhD, and Anne Marie O'Hanlon PhD at the University of New Orleans, who have laid the foundation for my scientific knowledge in the field of exercise physiology.

Bum Lee

We would like to send a special thank you to Brandon Fratto, Shelly Sharek, Mike Banach, and Erin Orahood. Although not featured in this book for technical reasons, they were kind enough to give their time and effort for its publication.

About the Authors

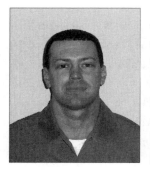

John Laurie is the co-founder and former CEO of Infinite Fitness Inc., a personal training company based solely on Human Resistance Training. He has developed training programs for high school, collegiate, and professional athletes. He is the co-founder of the Human Resistance Trainers Association (HRTA). Currently, Mr. Laurie lives in New Orleans, LA, writing and pursuing a Ph.D.

Bum Lee is co-owner of B.C. Power Factory, which specializes in custom leather athletic accessories. Formerly serving in the U.S. Marine Corps, Mr. Lee is the co-founder of the HRTA. He holds a BS in exercise physiology and has served as an athletic trainer for the University of New Orleans sports programs. He holds the Arkansas State AAU power lifting record for his weight class (165 lbs.) at 1,290 lbs.

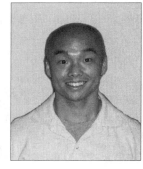

About the Models

Karynne Hoffman (left) is a graduate assistant at the University of New Orleans, where she is completing her Master's Degree in health care management. She works as an aerobics instructor and personal trainer at UNO. She is AFFA-certified and is a member of the National Institute for Recreation Sports Association (NIRSA).

Chris Grantner (second from left) is a part time fitness model. He is the co-founder of B.C. Power Factory, which specializes in custom leather athletic accessories.

Frances Hernandez (third from left) is a part-time model. She currently attends the University of New Orleans, majoring in Chemistry.

Monica Danby (right) is an AFFA-certified personal trainer and an Exercise Physiology major at the University of New Orleans.

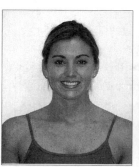

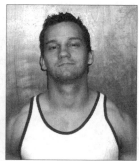

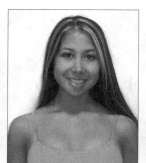

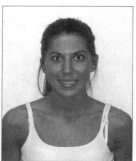

Table of Contents

1.

Introduction: What is Human Resistance Training?

If you have never heard the term Human Resistance Training (HRT) before, you may wonder what it means. In order to properly answer that question, we must first step backward and define resistance training. Technically, resistance training encompasses any type of exercise in which the human body works against a resistive force. If the definition sounds general, it is — and it needs to be because it covers a broad topic. Strength training with weights, machines, bands and tubing, calisthenics, HRT — all are forms of resistance training.

Human Resistance Training Explained

Human Resistance Training, or HRT, is a sub-category of resistance training and has far more narrow boundaries. By definition, HRT is any exercise in which the resistive force is provided only by another human being. As soon as another object, such as dumbbell, is introduced to provide resistance, the exercise no longer meets the definition of Human Resistance Training. There are of course, certain exceptions to this definition. Items such as lightweight bars, towels, and straps, which provide no significant weight themselves, but are used only to transfer the resistive force from one person to another are acceptable. This definition inevitably leads people to wonder if calisthenics (push ups, pull ups) are a form of Human Resistance Training. The answer is no, such exercises remain in the area of calisthenics until a second person (a partner) becomes the resistive force during the exercise.

Chances are, you have never heard of HRT (also known as Manual Resistance Training) up until now. Although little known, even to most people in the fitness and athletic fields, HRT is not new. Although its exact origins are not entirely clear, it has been used over the past century as a viable, low cost, training method. Until recently, most use of HRT has been limited to training in some foreign and domestic military units and the occasional athletic team. More prominently, the Air Force Academy football team has made use of HRT as a small but consistent part of their training regimen.

But why are so few people aware of HRT and even fewer use it? Up to this point HRT has consisted of only a small number of exercises, generally less than twenty although a few people claimed to have developed twenty-five to thirty. Such a small number of exercises means limitations in variety, and because many of these were single-joint exercises, it resulted in low sport specificity (as far as athletes are concerned). Additionally, the vast majority of the exercises were designed inefficiently, making it difficult for the

trainer to provide resistance and the participant to comfortably perform the exercise. The net effect has caused most people familiar with the concept to view it as interesting but only of limited value.

It was through these inherent and frustrating limitations that a breakthrough in the field of HRT was formed. While a dramatic increase in the number of exercises that could be performed was essential, this could not be accomplished until a higher level of efficiency was achieved. While a few of the exercises remain the same, others were reworked with special emphasis placed the laws of physics. Each exercise became incredibly efficient as physics was made to work for the trainer and participant. The foundation of nearly every exercise is the creation of a leverage advantage in favor of the trainer. In addition, the force of gravity is utilized, so that the trainer needs to expend only a minimal amount of energy in order to provide resistance to the participant that is far greater than could be achieved using muscle power alone. A significant benefit from this is two people of unequal size can now partner during HRT, which was not previously possible. As a result, the number of HRT exercises increased dramatically, and many exercises which could previously only be performed in a gym with equipment can now be performed nearly anywhere without equipment.

HRT requires no strength training equipment, but a partner is necessary in order to perform the exercises. While some view this as a disadvantage, it is actually advantageous because either partner can act as the trainer or participant, taking turns at getting the exercise. The trainer is much like a living, thinking, all-in-one, exercise

exercise efficiency, adaptability, and motivation are greatly increased. All of these of course are positive traits. However, people sometimes assume that because one person is generally referred to as the "trainer" (also called "spotter") and the other person is the "participant" (also called "client" or "performer") that special skills are necessary to take part. This is not the case. You do not need to be a personal trainer, have a degree in exercise physiology, or be a workout fanatic in order to use this system. A basic understanding of strength training — which is covered in this book, is all that is necessary. There is a learning curve, which is short, that occurs during the first few weeks of training. During this time, exercise performance efficiency will not be 100 percent, because the trainer is still learning how to use leverage and gravity to its full advantage. Fortunately, using HRT is much like riding a bike. The more you use it, the easier it gets.

There will always be people who are skeptical of this type of training. After all, it is difficult to imagine that many people who are seeking fitness benefits with equipment can attain the same results with training methods that do not use equipment. However, two points must be kept in mind. One, the exercises in this book are exactly the same as those done in the gym. They have the same movement, the same range of motion, and provide the same resistive force. Two, refer back to the original definition of resistance exercise. Resistive force is resistive force. The muscles of the body have no awareness of what is providing resistance to them as they work. Regardless of whether the resistive force is a metal weight, sand filled dumbbell, a log, or flesh and bone, the mus-

cular action is performed in the same way. Because of this, the applications of HRT are greatly increased. Many of the limitations that constrain traditional exercises are not present in HRT. Although not a cure-all by any means, HRT represents a step forward in the fields of fitness, athletics, and health.

Who Can Benefit from HRT?

Well, anybody, really. But here are some specifics about the benefits for different categories of people.

Athletes

Part of being an athlete is continually looking for ways to improve your performance, striving to get that "edge" which will separate you from you opponents. Most athletes (especially elite athletes) have already been exposed to nearly every type of exercise, including plyometrics, weight training, sport specific training and periodization techniques. Previously, HRT had little specificity to athletes because most of the few exercises which were available were single-joint movements. With the increase in the efficiency and number of exercises in this book, there is a far greater application for all sports. Some of the exercises can even be done with explosive movements, allowing for greater gains in power and speed, critical elements in all sports.

Personal Trainers

If you are a personal trainer, it is likely that you have already recognized the potential value of HRT to your business. Traditionally, personal trainers have had to work where the equipment has been — the fitness centers. In recent years almost all fitness centers have followed the universal trend of taking part of the money a trainer makes for every session with every client. The going rate is generally 25–30 percent of what the client is charged. A number of gyms have even gone so far as to require that the trainer works for the gym, allowing for a much larger cut of the profits, often up to 50 percent. Until now, trainers have been forced into this type of arrangement with little recourse. Traveling to a client's home required the trainer to bring his or her own weights. Time consuming and inefficient because you can only bring so much equipment with you, meaning the client will rapidly become stronger than the amount of weight you can adequately supply. Using HRT either exclusively or as a supplement eliminates this problem, allowing you to give a better workout wherever you want to, while keeping most if not all of the money you make.

People on a Budget

Most people do have the desire to get fit and stay in shape. Actually attaining good health and fitness is another matter. It is a shame but a number of people simply can't afford to get in shape by purchasing a gym membership which often costs 30 to 70 dollars a month and requires signing up for a year. Many who make the sacrifices to afford gym membership find themselves ill educated with regards to fitness. Usually, this leads to frustration, lack of results, and little use of an expensive membership. Purchasing a home gym requires much the same financial commitment, and more often than not, it becomes what has been called the "world's most expensive clothes rack." And hiring a personal trainer? For those who have difficulty affording the monthly membership dues in a commercial gym, the cost of hiring a personal trainer at $30–$70 per session is out of the question. This book illustrates and explains how an exercise is performed, providing not only a cost effective alternative but an applicable, exercise knowledge base as well.

Business Men and Women

Many times being part of the business world requires frequent travel and long hours. Business people are constantly on the run and fitness is often set on the back burner. Often, there is little time for lunch let alone a trip to the gym. Corporate travel has a tremendously negative impact on fitness. Most companies tend to economize business trips, attempting to get the best value for their dollar. Because of this, most business travelers end up staying at hotels with inadequate or no fitness rooms. While many hotels boast a "fitness center" as one of their amenities, closer inspection reveals the fitness center is usually a universal machine and a treadmill. With HRT, hotels don't need to have gyms. Exercise can be done in the space of the hotel room. This maximizes time and efficiency, two attributes which successful businesses rely on.

Coaches and Group Instructors

The dilemma of many physical education instructors, group instructors (military, police, etc.) and coaches is that there are many people and a limited supply of space and equipment. When budget cuts are made, physical education, fitness, and sports programs are usually the first ones to be cut. With only a few pieces of equipment meant to cover a wide range of exercises, some get to exercise while others have to wait. Certainly, not all of those who are working out are performing the same exercise. This makes supervision and instruction a problem. A coach or instructor cannot possibly keep tabs on everyone at the same time, watching form, technique, and making corrections. HRT is a cost effective way to teach and monitor small, medium, and large groups regardless of the ability and experience of those participating.

Anyone Seeking Fitness Alternatives

There are more than a few people out there looking for specific characteristics when joining a fitness center. Some are attracted to the social gym, with blaring techno music, overly zealous salespeople, and a host of other attributes which are detrimental to fitness. Many prefer the no-nonsense gym. You know the kind — big, sweaty men clanking heavy dumbbells around while grunting. There is of course, nothing wrong with this, but it can intimidate many people looking to join a gym. Other people are afraid of going to a gym and not knowing what to do or feeling self-conscious about the way they look. With HRT, you can partner up with someone you feel extremely comfortable with in the comfort of your own home. No need to worry about the pressures (real or conceived) of working out in a public setting. After all, getting results is far more difficult if you are worrying about other people and your surroundings rather than concentrating on the task at hand.

The Benefits of HRT

Compared to other forms of training, here are some of the major advantages of HRT.

Safety

Safety is a clear advantage of HRT over more conventional methods. When using free weights, there is always the danger, that no matter how experienced the lifter, that the weights may be dropped on the body causing injury. For example, during the bench press the bar (which weighs 45 lbs. alone) can get stuck on the chest or neck of the lifter when they cannot perform the final repetition to completion. There have even been a few incidents where dropped weights have caused the chest to collapse or the neck to be broken, (although these incidents are extremely rare) resulting in death. In HRT, the participant never has to worry about falling weights. The trainer acts simultaneously as the spotter and the weight, ensuring the highest level of safety. The trainer is in control of the speed and force of the resistance and can adjust either almost instantaneously. The trainer can provide smooth resistance during an isometric repetition or static contraction (the muscle is not lengthening or shortening, it is working by remaining still) for an isotonic repetition. If the participant is involved in athletic training, the trainer could implement a controlled, high velocity repetition, making the exercises more specific to the individual's sport, while maintaining a high level of safety. The resistance of any exercise will never exceed a dangerous speed in the control of a responsible trainer.

Cost and Space Effective

The majority of the exercises in this book require no equipment other than the human body. The exercises that do require equipment are demonstrated here using only a durable plastic bar. The bar is lightweight, approximately three feet long, and can stand up to the resistance of two individuals weighing up to 250 lbs. each. Other forms of HRT have used towels or belts, which work well, although we feel the bar is more versatile. By contest, gym memberships and home gyms are for more costly and tend to go unused by the purchaser.

Additionally, very little space is required for HRT. If two people can find enough space to fit into, it is likely they can perform the exercises in this book. Home gyms and similar equipment usually take up valuable floor space and are often difficult to move. Have you ever tried to lug gym equipment on a business trip or to the office? Chances are it was a noble, yet short lived experiment. The knowledge contained in this book allows for workouts every bit as effective, if not

more so, than training at a gym— at a fraction of the cost and/or space requirement.

Multiplicity

Most fitness centers have two or three of the most popular pieces of equipment in the gym and usually one of everything else. This is to enable them to cut down on space requirements as well as cost. Unfortunately, this might mean waiting in line to use that equipment for you. This problem is especially prevalent during the "peak" hours, usually before and after work or school. After a long day of work and fighting traffic trying to get to the gym, the last thing you want to do is wait ten or fifteen minutes for a piece of equipment to open up. Few things kill motivation or training technique faster. If you are a coach or involved in team sports, it can be difficult to train the entire team at once using limited equipment unless the team's sponsoring organization has an unlimited budget. With HRT, literally hundreds of athletes can be trained at once, as long as there is an even number of people (one trainer, one participant).

Adaptability

The human muscle adapts to stressors (such as exercises) by getting stronger and larger. When performing an exercise such as biceps curls, the muscles are broken down at the cellular level, causing microscopic tears in the muscle. This is why you get sore after exercising. If you continue to do biceps curls over and over again, the muscles will stop adapting and you will no longer see the same results. The human muscle can adapt to any exercise if done often enough, because it goes through the same motion with the maximum and minimum stresses occurring at the same times at the same locations.

A muscle may be able to adjust to an inert weight or machine, but this is nearly impossible using HRT. With free weights or machines, maximum stress is not always continuously placed on the muscle. As the muscles rotate the weights from point A to point B, the resistance lever gets shorter or longer. This means that maximum stress is only obtained during one point in the exercise movement. Because the trainer is providing the weight, resistance can be manipulated by placing more stress when the resistance arm is short and decreasing the amount of stress when the resistance arm is long. This allows variable force at different points during the exercise, ensuring maximum stress is obtained at more than one portion of the movement. In short, the trainer becomes a thinking, reactive exercise machine, capable of rapid adjustments, ensuring high level results.

Transfer of Knowledge

HRT uniquely helps to facilitate the knowledge of the mechanics of exercise. The two-person system works like a series of checks and balances. If the exercise is being done with incorrect form, both the client and the trainer will be able to feel that the movement is incorrect. In this way, both the participant and the trainer learn proper form and technique, which can be carried over to other forms of strength training.

Each of the exercise's movements done with HRT are exactly the same as those performed in a gym with machines and free weights. The only difference is the way in which the resistance is provided (human vs. metal). Because of this, learning proper form and technique through HRT allows someone who has never lifted weights before to go to a gym and perform the same exercises using equipment. Conversely, the same is true for someone who uses gym equipment but has never done HRT.

Equipment

Although it might seem a bit odd to have a section on equipment in a book about exercising without strength training equipment, there are actually some auxiliary devices used to transfer the resistive force to the participant. They act as conduits through which the resistance flows. Not all are needed for each exercise, although two human beings are the constant in HRT.

The Human Machine

The human body is a remarkable, complex machine, with perhaps its greatest asset being adaptability. This adaptability allows us to complete a seemingly endless variety of tasks, from the simple and mundane to the delicate and complex. Many of the exercises in this book take advantage of this. With HRT, the human body is the equipment. Think of it as a living, thinking, all in one piece of strength training equipment — for that is exactly what it is.

The Bar

Some of the exercise designed for this book require the use of a bar or rod to effectively duplicate the motions of machines and weights found in fitness centers and gyms. The bar itself, made of a strong, lightweight plastic, contains almost no weight itself (approx. 2 lbs.) and does not add any noticeable resistive force.

Miscellaneous Objects

Previous HRT exercises made use of items such as towels or belts in order to transfer resistance from the trainer to the participant. Although we chose to use a plastic bar instead, everyday items such as towels and belts demonstrate the adaptability of HRT, showing that it can be done nearly anywhere with very little or no resources. Because HRT is a highly adaptable form of training, other objects, such as stairs, chairs, couches, or any stable platform can be used to exercise. As long as the angles are correct, leverage is present, and safety is ensured, HRT can be augmented with a variety of objects, which do not provide resistance themselves.

Terminology

Throughout this book, we have used the terms "participant" and "trainer" to refer to the person doing the exercise and the second person respectively. As explained elsewhere in this chapter, the roles are interchangeable, so each partner can get a turn at exercise and at providing the resistance. If you are applying these exercises in the capacity of personal trainer, feel free to read "client" instead of "participant." Conversely, if you prefer to think in a more informal context, you may refer to the "trainer" as "spotter" or "helper."

2.

The Dynamics of Human Resistance Training

In this chapter, we'll be exploring the interactions, relationships, responsibilities, and procedures that are important in HRT methods. As explained in the preceding chapter, we'll be referring to the person carrying out the exercise as the "participant" and the one providing the resistance as the "trainer" in order to keep the responsibilities of the two parties clearly defined.

Responsibilities of the Trainer

Communication

It is important that the trainer is in constant communication with the participant, especially during the initial stages of exercise. The trainer is likely to be unfamiliar with the participant's strength at

first. Talking throughout the entire exercise, gaining as much information from the participant as possible is crucial to HRT. As well as verbal communication, the trainer should do his or her best to pick up on non-verbal cues the participant is sending out.

The trainer's eyes should constantly be on the participant; looking for any signs of improper form, fatigue, distress, discomfort, or injury. The trainer has the optimal view of the movement, and should be constantly making adjustments to the exercise. During the initial stages of the exercises, the trainer should try to learn the habits of the participant. The more quickly a trainer can gather information and respond, the more likely the participant is to have a safe, productive training session.

Safety

HRT is not designed for a one rep maximum test, nor is it a testing ground for potentially dangerous movements. The safety of the participant is in the trainer's hands. It is not important for the trainer to bear as much weight as they can for the first couple of repetitions, unless the participant is just that strong. Loading all the weight on the participant for the first repetition can also cause a real unsteadiness or even injury to both the trainer and the participant.

Remember, during the course of the exercises the trainer and the participant are partners. The participant relies on the trainer for his or her safety and health. Breaching the trust between training partners renders HRT nearly useless. Although the potential for injury always exists during any type of exercise, the participant must remain confident that the trainer is able to provide the maximum level of safety.

Provide Variable Resistance

The human skeletal and muscular system is a complex system of levers. So therefore, the laws of physics are constantly at work. Using the laws of physics, Human Resistance exercises are designed to allow the trainer a maximum amount of leverage. This allows the trainer to do comparatively little work in order to provide a great deal of resistance to the participant. It is up to the trainer (based on a number of factors) to decide how much resistance to provide.

Because the trainer is able to make adjustments, it is possible to provide maximum resistance to the participant at every point in his or her range of motion — something that is impossible using free weights. As the eccentric motion nears completion, slightly reduce the amount of resistance, allowing the participant to fully contract the muscles. During the eccentric motion, when the muscles are strongest (up to 140 percent of the weight of a concentric movement can be lifted) it is probable that more force will have to be provided to the participant. Be careful however. It is common during the first few weeks of training to experience a learning curve in which the trainer has a tendency to use too little or too much weight at certain points. This can easily be overcome by proper communication between the trainer and participant.

Responsibilities of the Participant

Communication

The participant must always maintain communication with the trainer. The participant's safety and effectiveness of the workout depend on it. Unbalanced positioning, too much leverage, not enough leverage, or a bad angle of resistance can lead to injury for both the participant and the trainer. The participant and trainer should first experiment with the positioning and use light resistance to begin with and increase the leverage and the force after talking it over. Clear communication must be established with every exercise until a smooth and steady movement and resistance are established. Don't be afraid to speak up. Please refer to the section of this book on Communication and the HRT Fatigue Scale.

Consistency of Movement

It is important to make sure that the movement is steady throughout the duration of the exercise. Sudden loss of tension, especially if the trainer is unaware that it is about to occur, is dangerous. This could lead to a loss of balance, potential fall (depending on the exercise), or strains and sprains for both you and the trainer. In general, smaller, gradual, lapses in tension are common during exercise. This most often occurs as the muscles go from the concentric to eccentric movement, often without the participant even realizing it. It is likely that the trainer will notice any loss of tension and make you aware of it, but it is always a good idea to keep this thought at the forefront of your consciousness.

Achieve Maximum Contraction

At the completion of the concentric motion and again at the completion of the eccentric motion, it is important to squeeze the muscle and pause slightly. By pausing in the contracted position,

the muscles are able to develop maximally throughout the entire range of motion. Achieving maximum contraction also benefits you by helping to ensure a steady movement and tension throughout the exercise. Pausing allows you to avoid a bouncing or ballistic motion at the beginning of each concentric and eccentric phase, which causes a break in the movement and reduces the effectiveness of the exercise.

Maximum Effort

Always exert the maximum amount of effort (in a controlled manner) when performing an exercise. Be sure to perform all exercises to temporary muscle fatigue. Half efforts will produce little to no results, regardless of the training method or style. When using conventional strength training equipment such as machines or free weights, you are the only one who knows whether or not you gave it your all. This is not the case with HRT.

The trainer can literally feel whether or not you are giving maximum effort in response to the resistance. Of course you could try to take it easy during the workout but you would only be cheating yourself. Chances are, the trainer will lose patience and interest quickly if you decide not to work hard.

Cooperation

Cooperation between the participant and trainer are crucial. As the participant, you need to remember that it is not a contest between you and the trainer to see who is the strongest. The vast majority of the time the trainer can overpower the participant because of the leverage and gravity advantages each exercise provides. The participant can however make life more difficult for the trainer at certain points during the exercise by stopping or changing form. Turning the exercise into a grudge match is an invitation to injury or at the very least, a waste of time. Think of the trainer as a piece of equipment and perform the exercise as you would in the gym.

Communication

Communication is a lynch pin in the concept and practice of HRT. While the trainer is able to pick up on the physical cues displayed by the participant's muscles and body language, a verbal give and take is also an important part of the process. One reason is the issue of safety. The participant should be readily able to recognize the difference between the burning sensation, which occurs as the muscle fatigues, and sharp localized pain, which is most often indicative of injury. The participant should always speak up if they suspect injury, in which case the exercise would stop, or improper form or technique, so adjustments can be made during the course of the exercise

The second reason of the importance of communication is that it directly relates to performance when using HRT. It is the trainer's responsibility to continually ask the participant questions during the course of the exercise, attempting to gauge the participant's perception of how much work is being done by the muscle, how much fatigue has set in, and that the muscles being worked are the ones intended. In this way the trainer is able to "adjust" the weight during the exercise, tailoring the resistance level provided to the fatigue level of the participant's muscles. While it is true that neither the trainer nor the participant knows exactly how much "weight" (e.g. 50 lbs.) is being provided during the course of the exercise, non-verbal communication and the use of the HRT Fatigue Scale (explained on pages 22 and 23) helps to make this traditional stumbling block a virtual non-issue.

Non-Verbal Communication

Non-verbal communication is present in any traditional gym setting as well as nearly every athletic endeavor. The most obvious non-verbal cues are fairly easy to pick out. The weight lifter attempting to get that last repetition may exhibit shaking muscles, a change in form, or holding his or her breath as they struggle to finish. Even sitting at home watching a your favorite team play, you can pick up non-verbal cues. As the game wears on did you notice the running back favor one leg, or the basketball player stand upright instead of getting down into proper defensive position? These are non-verbal indicators of potential injury and fatigue.

When using HRT, the importance of non-verbal communication takes on a central role. During every single exercise the trainer is in direct contact with the participant. Through the movement of the exercise the trainer is able to feel exactly what the participant's muscles are doing. The trainer can feel if the movement is smooth or slightly shaky, if the current amount of resistance provided is too little, if one body part is favored over another (improper form), changes in form, and the decrease in muscular strength as the client's muscles continue to work.

An immense amount of information is transmitted from the participant to the trainer instantaneously, as the movement of the exercise occurs. This allows the trainer to make on the spot adjustments necessary to maximize the effectiveness of the workout. Essentially, the trainer becomes a thinking, reactive exercise machine, capable of quickly increasing or decreasing resistance, adjusting form, torque, angles, and the amount of repetitions in order to efficiently complete the exercise for the highest possible level of effectiveness.

But what adjustment should be made and when? This is a standard question. In order to take a great deal of guesswork out of HRT, five common scenarios are listed below with their probable causes and solutions. These scenarios are listed as the trainer would "feel" them through the course of the exercise.

Scenario

1. The movement feels "jerky" or "broken up"; not smooth and controlled as an exercise done with equipment would feel.

   ■ Check your grip. Either the trainer or the participant, or both may be gripping tightly during the exercise. Most exercises require a relatively open or lose grip. Tightening your grip commonly causes the movement to become unstable.

   ■ Make sure the participant is not trying to "overpower" the trainer during the exercise. Remind the participant to use a smooth controlled motion, as if they were using a piece of equipment.

   ■ Make sure the trainer is not trying to "overpower" the participant. This may be an indication of too much resistance being applied by the trainer.

2. The participant struggles through the movement to the point of not being able to properly complete the exercise.

   ■ The trainer may not be making the necessary adjustments as the participant fatigues. Remember, the trainer is like an adjustable piece of exercise equipment. As the participant fatigues, lighten up slightly to allow a complete movement.

3. The participant rushes easily through the exercise or takes and especially high number of repetitions to fatigue.

   ■ It is likely that the trainer is not applying enough resistance in this case, most likely from the outset of the movement. Don't be afraid to apply resistance to the participant, you can always lighten the load.

   ■ If the participant does not continue to fatigue after a certain point during the exercise, chances are the trainer has overcompensated by decreasing the amount of resistance unknowingly or decreasing the amount of resistance a little too much as the participant worked toward complete muscle fatigue.

4. The participant feels a different muscle group working than the one the exercise is supposed to work.

■ In this case the angle used during the setup is not correct causing other muscles to perform during the movement. The trainer should check the exercise in the book to ensure the proper angle and alignment is used. Most exercise require a 45-degree angle at the lever. Deviation from this angle usually causes the problem.

5. The trainer feels as if they are getting as much of a workout during the exercise as the participant.

■ This is common among people who are new to HRT. It is a natural reaction to try and provide resistance for the participant by using your own muscle power. Try to relax and let gravity and your own body weight do the work for you. Almost all of the exercises are designed so the trainer has the leverage advantage, so little muscle power is needed. Keep practicing!

Verbal Communication

Verbal response during HRT is the second component of communication. While either non-verbal or verbal communication could theoretically be used exclusively during exercise, it is always a good idea to combine the use of both. Verbal communication is valuable because it gives the trainer an idea of the participant's direct perceptions of what they are experiencing. In order to enhance the value of verbal communication during HRT and to help tailor the workout to the individual, we developed the HRT Fatigue Scale, to help the participant to best communicate what they are feeling. The scale allows for little guesswork and helps ensure both the trainer and the participant are on the same page at all times during the workout.

The HRT Fatigue Scale is a verbal indicator of the participant's muscle fatigue. The trainer should ask what level the participant is at every two to three repetitions. This allows the trainer to adjust the amount of resistance placed on the participant accordingly. This continues throughout the duration of the exercise until the participant reaches temporary muscle fatigue.

The HRT Fatigue Scale

The HRT Fatigue Scale, shown in the box on the facing page, is a primary communicative tool between the trainer and the participant. The scale has five different levels associated with the level of muscle fatigue or "burn" associated with any given exercise. A probable communication between the trainer and participant during exercise would go as follows:

■ Trainer: "What Level?"

■ Participant: "Three"

At this point, the trainer makes an assessment of the participant's condition. The participant has indicated "3" (meaning Level 3) as his or her perception of muscle fatigue during the exercise. The trainer understands this to mean that muscle "burn" has started to occur and the participant is working toward "burnout" on that particular muscle.

The trainer takes in the participant's perception of muscular work as well as how the participant's muscles "feel" during the exercise. The trainer can then make an accurate judgment as to how much muscular endurance is left, whether to increase or decrease the amount of resistance being provided and the amount of strength the participant has gained over time. By asking at what level the participant is at every few repetitions, the trainer is able to make on the spot adjustments to tailor the workout to the individual.

Hand Positioning and Grip

Hand positioning and grip is of key importance in every single HRT exercise that is performed. Because HRT relies on one individual manually providing resistance to another, where and how the trainer's hands are placed help determine the efficiency and effectiveness of the participant's performance. The trainer's hand position in relation to the participant serves as the point of contact through which leverage, torque, and resistance form the exercise.

Hand positioning and grip can be thought of as the connecting piece of two interlocking machines. If the connection is off, either one or both of the machines cannot perform their function properly. Improper positioning may shorten or lengthen the lever arm, resulting in a movement that is very difficult to administer for the trainer and difficult to complete for the participant. The

The HRT Fatigue Scale	
Stage	**Descriptive Features**
Level 1	Relatively Docile, Little Muscular Action Taking Place
Level 2	Muscle Begins to Perform, Slight Muscle Fatigue Present
Level 3	Muscle Burn is Present, Significant Muscular Work
Level 4	Significant Muscle Burn, Increasing Toward Fatigue
Level 5	Muscle Burnout, Complete Muscle Fatigue

resulting lack of efficiency in either resistance or movement can have detrimental effects on the participant. If the resistance point is incorrect, it is likely that the participant will not be able to work the muscle group intended during the exercise, in a worst case scenario, resulting in injury. Listed below are hand grip and positioning techniques, demonstrating proper form.

Hand to Body

When the trainer places his or her hands on a part of the participant's body, the position of greatest effectiveness is near the joint furthest from the axis of rotation. This creates the greatest amount of leverage to provide resistance. Hand placement should be just above the joint but not over it, which could cause injury. Always use a flat open palm grip, which ensures a steady,

smooth movement. The picture above shows proper positioning during side lateral raises.

Hand to Hand

Certain exercises require the trainer to interlock hands with the participant. Hand positions differ from exercise to exercise and are explained on the exercise description page of each. As a general rule, the trainer's and the participant's hands should come together at the palms of the hands. The grip should be firm enough to stay inter-

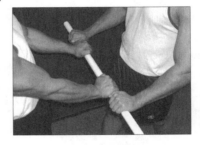

Top left: Fig. 2.3. Correct hand position.

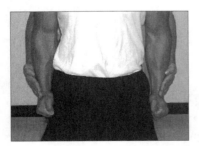

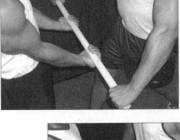

Above: Fig. 2.1. Correct side raise hand position.
Right: Fig. 2.2. Incorrect side raise hand position.

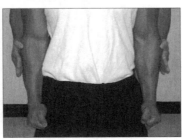

Above and right: Figs. 2.4 and 2.5. Incorrect hand positions.

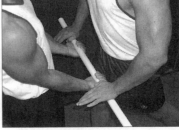

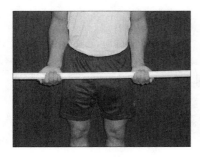

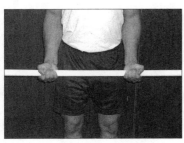

Above: Fig. 2.6. Correct hand position.
Right: Fig. 2.7. Incorrect hand position.

Bar Grip

For exercises that require the use of a bar, the trainer has less of a margin of error. The bar creates an additional interface between the trainer and the participant. Because of this, improper hand position or grip can more easily destabilize the movement. The trainer's hands are positioned exactly the same during every exercise that requires the bar.

The trainer should place his or her hands immediately outside the hands of the participant, so that they are almost touching. The grip should be open-palmed or lightly closed, with the bar resting in the palms of the trainer's hands. Although some of the exercises may require a variation of this type of grip (and are described with the exercise), the open palm grip allows for the greatest level of ease through the movement. Take a minute to work through all of the types of grips, including incorrect ones, pictured in this section. It becomes apparent how difficult and inefficient the exercises become when proper grip is not maintained.

locked and maintain a smooth, steady movement. A harder grip can cause an uneven motion during the exercise, a softer one could cause a loss of grip, resulting in a break in the movement and possible injury. Figure 2.1 on the facing page shows the proper grip during 1-arm lateral pulls.

3.

Foundations of Exercise

This chapter will explore the basic concepts and the various factors that come into play in HRT. Once again, not all of this is specific only to HRT alone but is common to all exercise methods. However, since these principles are important, and since we can't be sure all readers are aware of them, they are covered in some detail here.

Strength Training Basics

This section briefly overviews basic concepts in strength training, primarily geared toward HRT and the exercises presented in this book. No attempt is made to present training programs or cycles due to the wide range of people HRT applies to. The areas covered here are purposefully general. While it is not essential to have knowledge or expertise in fitness in order to use

HRT, basic concepts are necessary in order to correctly and effectively develop strength training programs. Because of this, the concepts that are presented here may not necessarily apply to advanced fitness participants or to athletes using sport specific exercise and periodization models.

Muscular Contractions

In the context of this book, muscular contractions fall into three categories: isometric, concentric, and eccentric. Isometric contractions, also known as static contractions occur when a specific muscle group performs work against a resistive force without changing length. For example, one exercise in this book is isometric — the wall squat. During the exercise, the participant remains in a fixed position while the quadriceps work against the force of gravity until exhaustion. Isometric contractions generally have much less value in terms of functional strength, especially to athletes, than concentric or eccentric contractions.

Concentric and eccentric contractions tend to occur during the same exercise movement. The concentric movement, also known as the "positive" movement occurs as the muscle shortens against a resistive force. An example is the lifting phase of the chest press, when the weight is pressed (lifted) from the chest. Eccentric movement, also known as the "negative" movement occurs as the muscle lengthens against a resistive force. For an example we refer back to the chest press. As the weight is lowered back toward the chest, the muscle lengthens against the force of resistance. Eccentric strength can be up to 140 percent of concentric strength and are primarily responsible for microscopic tears in muscle fiber, resulting in increased strength.

Exercise Order

The order in which you choose to do your exercises must be carefully considered. In general, optimal results will be more readily attained if the large muscle groups (legs, chest, back) are exercised before smaller muscle groups (shoulders, triceps, biceps). The reasoning behind this is simple. You want the larger muscle groups to be able to perform as much work as possible. No muscle group works independently, all are associated in one way or another with other muscle groups. For example, almost every chest exercise requires using the triceps (back of the arms) to some degree. If you were to exercise your triceps (a smaller muscle group) before your chest (a large muscle group), it is unlikely you would be

Table 3.1. Ways you can help prevent and alleviate muscle soreness

Preventing Soreness	Alleviating Soreness
Warm up thoroughly before strength training.	Warm up the body with light aerobic work, calisthenics, or light stretching sore muscles.
Stretch completely after training.	Take a mild anti-inflammatory (e.g. aspirin or ibuprofen). *
Make sure you get enough vitamins and minerals.	Take a long, hot bath.

* Always consult a physician

able to exercise your chest completely to fatigue. Because the triceps work in an auxiliary fashion for most chest exercises, fatiguing them first would ensure they would fatigue again, and more quickly than the chest during a chest exercise. Additionally, multi-joint exercises are performed before single-joint exercises in the same muscle group (for example, power squats before leg extensions).

Other important considerations to be made when determining exercise order is the fitness level of the participant and the purpose of the training routine. Giant sets (two or more consecutive exercises for the same muscle) are most likely too much for the beginner's body to handle. There is significant risk of increased, prolonged muscle soreness as well as the possibility of injury. Athletes on the other hand, who are training for a specific purpose, might purposely use giant sets, supersets, and other methods more advanced than those seeking different results.

Muscle Soreness

If you put effort into your training, you can expect some soreness, especially in the beginning. Soreness is part of the body's adaptive response to the stresses of exercise. Tiny, microscopic tears in the muscle fiber, as a result of exercise, cause the soreness to occur. The cellular damage signals the body to repair muscle tissue and make it stronger than before.

Muscle soreness is nothing to fear; you just need to treat it as a signal from the body. Soreness indicates that you have challenged muscle

groups beyond their previous ability, which means they are recovering and improving. Slight soreness that occurs 24-48 hours after exercise is called Delayed Onset Muscle Soreness (DOMS). DOMS is characteristic of eccentric movements during exercise, which is primarily responsible for tears in the muscle fiber. If your muscles display symptoms such as acute localized soreness, lack of range of motion, and tenderness, and/or the soreness lasts beyond two days, you have trained a little too hard. Your body was not yet ready for this level of work. You will recover, but continued exercise without proper recovery will eventually lead to overtraining and a reversal of any gains you might make.

There are several ways you can help prevent and alleviate muscle soreness, as shown in Table. 3.1 on the facing page.

General Points

Strength Training

■ Perform the movement slowly and steadily. Don't suddenly release muscle tension or drop back to the starting position.

■ Pay special attention to the eccentric motion, also called the negative. Perform the eccentric motion in a controlled manner, helping to achieve muscle fatigue and optimum results.

■ Do as many repetitions as possible with proper form.

- Concentrate on the muscle group that is performing work during exercise.

- Never hold your breath while strength training, breath in a regular, consistent fashion.

- If you feel lightheaded, dizzy or nauseous, stop.

Cardiovascular Work

- When involved in any type of cardiovascular training (jumping jacks, running, aerobics, etc.), be sure to keep your knees relaxed and ready to bend with impact.

- Breathe deeply and as rapidly as necessary.

- Be sure to try as hard in cardiovascular aspects as you do in strength training.

- Stop if you feel lightheaded, dizzy, or nauseous.

Stretching

- Stretching speeds your recovery and development as well as preventing soreness and injury.

- Perform stretches smoothly and consistently, never bounce on a stretch.

- Stretch as far as you comfortably can and then try to maintain that position for 15–30 seconds.

- Always stretch after exercise.

Physics, Leverage, and Gravity

The human muscular and skeletal system is a highly symmetrical system of levers, so therefore, the laws of Torque are always present. The definition of Torque, or T, is the magnitude of force multiplied by the lever arm ($T = F \times L$). The line of action in which the direction of the force is being placed determines the Force F. The lever arm L is the distance between the line of action and the axis of rotation, measured on a line that is

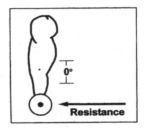

$T = F \times L$
$T = 45N \times (1m \times \sin 90)$
$T = 45Nm$

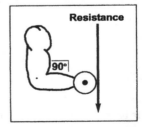

$T = F \times L$
$T = 45N \times (1m \times \sin 90)$
$T = 45Nm$

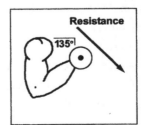

$T = F \times L$
$T = 45N \times (1m \times \sin 90)$
$T = 45Nm$

Fig. 3.1. Stress cycle during free weight exercise cycle.

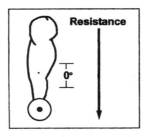
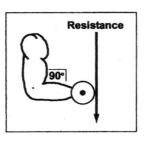
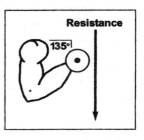

Fig. 3.2. Stress cycle during the same exercise using HRT.

T = F x L
T = 45N x (1m x sin 180)
T = 0Nm

T = F x L
T = 45N x (1m x sin 90)
T = 45Nm

T = F x L
T = 45N x (1m x sin 45)
T =31.82Nm

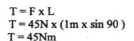

perpendicular to both (which is needed to put maximum stress on the muscle).

When using free weights, gravity is always pulling the weight down toward the ground. As the muscle is going through the range of motion, the resistance lever is becoming shorter or longer. The resistance lever never stays at its longest possible length throughout the movement (The resistance lever is longest when the resistance is perpendicular to the resistance arm). This creates a 90-degree angle between the resistance arm and the direction of the force. In order to achieve maximum muscle fiber recruitment, the muscle must be placed under constant pressure. This cannot happen if the resistance arm is constantly changing lengths and relieving stress from the muscle.

With HRT, the laws of Torque can be manipulated by changing the direction of the resistance. The trainer is able to compensate; adjusting the torque by increasing the amount of pressure as the resistance arm becomes longer or shorter, ensuring continuous resistance on the muscle.

This can be illustrated using the biceps curl as an example. As the participant begins the exercise, the lever arm starts at an angle of 0 degrees,

so the amount of torque is 0. As the forearm begins to rotate upward, the angle begins to rise toward 90 degrees. As the weight reaches 90 degrees maximal stress is placed on the muscle. Continuing through the motion passed 90 degrees, the stress is decreased once again. Fig. 3.1 illustrates this situation.

Fig. 3.2 shows the same exercise done using HRT. Instead of beginning at an angle of 0 degrees, the angle between the lever arm and the line of action can start at 90 degrees and remain there throughout the duration of the movement. This allows for maximal stress on the muscle during the entire movement.

Fitness Terminology

Throughout this book some terms will be used with which the reader may not be familiar, though these are common concepts in the field of fitness training. For those unfamiliar with this terminology, we have compiled a Glossary of Terms, which can be found in the Appendix at the end of the book, starting on page 161.

4.

Introduction to the Exercises

The following chapters contain about fifty HRT exercises as well as four aerobic exercises, divided over ten chapters, each dealing with a specific set of muscles, a specific part of the body, or (in Chapter 14), a specific type of exercise. In this introductory chapter, you will find general guidelines for the process of HRT as they will be applied in those exercises.

Each of the exercises depends on two human components, whom we refer to as trainer and participant respectively. The term trainer refers specifically to the person who administers resistance during the exercise. The trainer can also be referred to as the spotter or the partner.

No special qualifications or expertise are necessary in order to assume the role of the trainer, although it is important to carefully follow the instructions and pictures associated with each

individual exercise. The term participant refers to the individual actually performing the exercises. The participant can also be referred to as the lifter, athlete, or partner, and no prior fitness experience is necessary to perform the exercises.

It is important to understand that both the trainer and participant can and should function as independent, interchangeable, parts. Everyone who acts as the trainer or participant is encouraged to frequently switch roles. By doing this, each can learn how the movements work from the opposite perspective, and what is necessary to perform efficiently during exercise. As a result, the learning process becomes easier and the learning curve becomes shorter.

Exercise Page Setup

Each exercise description consists of one page of pictures, which move through the movement of the exercise from beginning stance to completion. The opposite page contains a written description

of how to perform the exercise, which corresponds to the pictures. The description page contains three sections and is set up in the following way:

Introduction

The introduction contains a brief description of the exercise. It includes the primary and secondary muscle groups, which perform the exercise, and the type of movement.

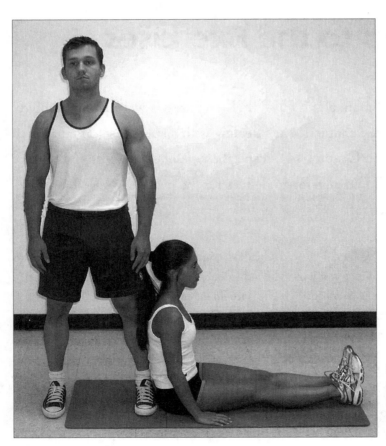

Fig. 4.1. Setup position for participant (seated) and trainer (standing) for exercises requiring setup. See text on facing page (p. 35) for details.

Trainer/Participant Position

This section has two parts. The first part describes the participant's starting position, distances, and angles necessary to perform the exercise. The second part describes the trainer's position in relation to the participant, the points at which resistance is applied to the participant, and the use of leverage and gravity.

The Movement

The movement describes how the exercise is performed from the start through completion, with information about range of motion, angle of rotation, and leverage.

Setup

Some exercises require the trainer and the participant to arrange themselves into a support position before the exercise begins. This is necessary for the support and protection of the participant's back, as well as stability and exercise efficiency. Each exercise that requires this position will contain a note in the Trainer/Participant Position section of the written description. The description will accompany each exercise although the picture (Fig. 4.1) will not.

Setup Position

The participant begins by sitting on the floor, with an upright posture and straight back. The trainer takes position behind the participant in a perpendicular fashion, so that the side of the trainer's leg and foot are flat against the center of the participant's back. With the alternate leg, the trainer steps back slightly, creating a solid base for the balance and support of the participant's back. The participant should maintain this posture, with the back straight and chest out for the duration of the exercise.

Exercises Requiring Setup

Here is a list of the exercises described in subsequent chapters that require this type of setup procedure. Please refer to these descriptions and illustration 4.1 for each of these exercises.

- Military Press

- Dumbbell Shoulder Press

- Half Arnold

- Overhead Triceps Extension

- Incline Bench Press*

- Dumbbell Incline Press*

---

* Exercises which require the trainer to take an additional step outward in order to create a 45- to 65-degree angle for the participant.

5.

Exercises for the Legs

The legs comprise two muscle groups which act as opposing forces: the knee extensors and the knee flexors. The knee extensor is the quadriceps group or upper front of the leg; the knee flexor is made up of the hamstring group (the back of the upper leg). Like the upper arm, the hamstrings are designed more for speed due to its muscle fiber arrangement. Conversely, the quadriceps are designed more for strength. It is important not to neglect the hamstring group to avoid damage of the knee joint.

In this and the following chapters, the relevant exercises for each muscle group will be covered by means of illustrations and a descriptive text on the opposing page. Here is a list of exercises contained in this chapter:

- Power squat
- Assisted squat

- Double leg extension
- Single leg extension
- Wall squat
- Lunges
- Hamstring curl
- Lying leg raise
- Seated calf raise

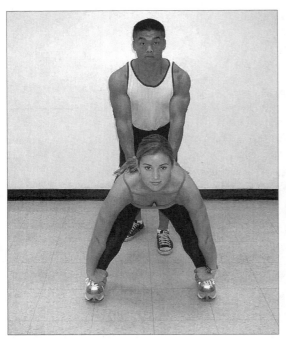
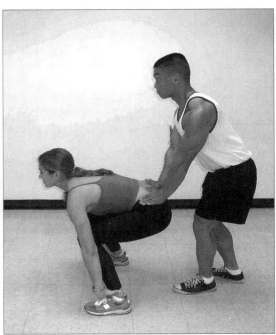

Fig. 5.1. Power squat. Above: starting position. Below: finishing position.

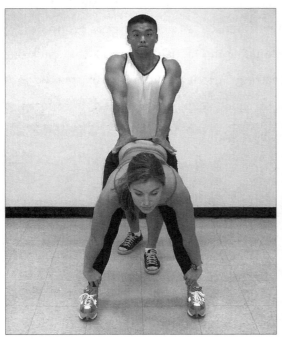
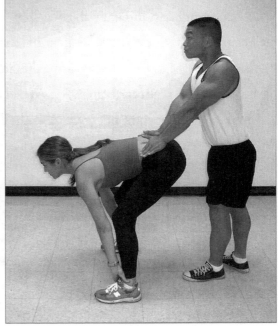

Power Squat

Introduction

- Primary muscles: hamstrings (back of the upper leg), and glutes (buttocks)

- Secondary muscles: quadriceps (front of the upper leg), and calves (back of the lower leg)

- Movement: multi-joint

- Performed: simultaneously with both legs

Trainer/Participant Position

Beginning in a standing stance, the participant positions his or her feet slightly further than shoulder-width apart, with the toes pointed slightly outward. Squatting down, the participant grabs the inside of each ankle with the corresponding hand. The back should be parallel to the floor in this position. The back should remain flat and the chin should remain up so the participant is looking forward during the movement.

The trainer takes position directly behind the participant, who is in the squatting position. Leaning down slightly, the trainer places his or her hands directly on or slightly below the hips of the participant. To avoid a loss of balance or injury to the participant, the trainer should be precise in hand placement. The trainer's feet are positioned shoulder-width apart, in an offset stance.

The Movement

The participant, starting in the squatting position, straightens the legs as much as possible while maintaining hand placement just above the ankles. During the eccentric phase, the participant slowly returns to the starting position, resisting the trainer. To avoid injury, the back should remain flat throughout the movement. The exercise is completed when the participant reaches fatigue.

The trainer provides resistance by pressing directly downward in a controlled manner. The same holds true during the eccentric phase of the exercise. The trainer creates leverage during this exercise by placing his or her body close to the participant's body, acting as a force multiplier. The trainer does not have to exert heavy pressure to achieve adequate resistance. Moving the body closer to the participant, with the chest over the participant's buttocks can increase resistance. The trainer should keep constant steady pressure and be sure the participant maintains proper foot, hand, and back positioning.

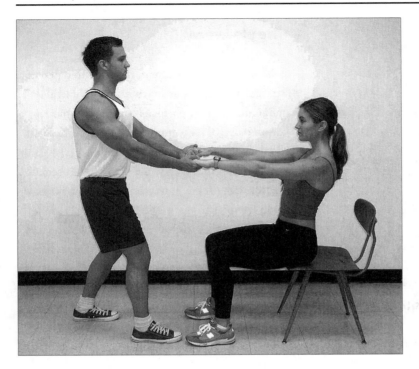

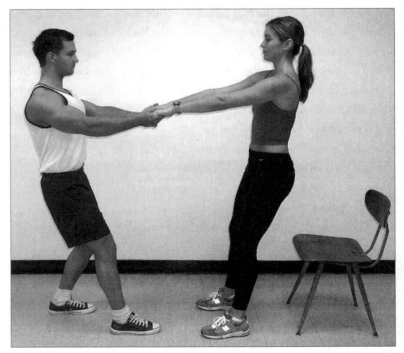

Fig. 5.2. Assisted squat.
Above: starting position.
Right: finishing position.

Assisted Squat

Introduction

- Primary muscle: quadriceps (front of the upper leg)

- Secondary muscles: hamstrings (back of the upper leg), gluteus (buttocks)

- Movement: multi-joint

- Performed: both legs simultaneously

Trainer/Participant Position

The participant begins the exercise by sitting on the edge of a sturdy chair or platform. The feet are positioned flat on the floor, shoulder-width apart. In this position, the participant's legs should form a 90-degree angle. The participant then extends the arms forward until they are parallel to the floor. The participant's back remains straight and the chest out for the duration of the exercise.

The trainer takes position by standing in front of the participant, at arm length from the participant's extended hands. The trainer's feet should be positioned in an offset stance, with one slightly in front of the other, about shoulder-width apart. This provides a strong base for the participant and maintains balance during the exercise. Reaching forward, the trainer firmly grasps the participant's hands.

The Movement

At the start of the exercise, the participant should extend his or her arms straight out toward the trainer and keep them in a loose, fixed position throughout the movement. The trainer holds the participant's hands firmly for support. The participant's arms remain straight and relaxed throughout the duration of the exercise. The participant then leans slightly backward while sitting in the chair. This will maintain resistance on the quadriceps during the movement. The participant then slowly rises to a standing position. During the eccentric phase, the participant slowly returns to the seated position.

The trainer maintains a firm hold of the participant's hands and counterbalances the weight of the participant to hold them up and avoid falling. The trainer may have to lean backward slightly to counterbalance the participant. Resistance is provided by the participant's own body weight, and the exercise is completed when the participant can no longer rise from the chair.

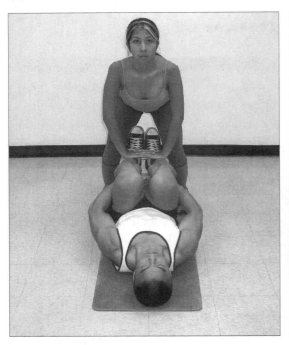
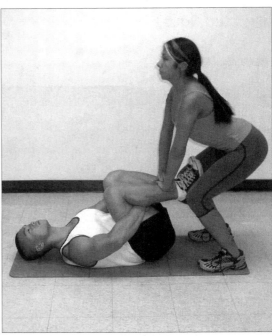

Fig. 5.3. Double leg extensions. Above: starting position. Below: finishing position.

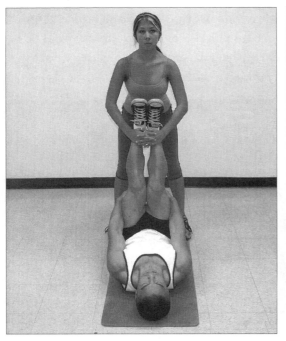
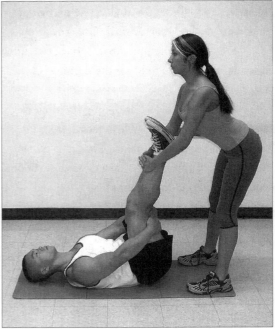

Double Leg Extension

Introduction

- Primary muscle: quadriceps

- Secondary muscle: not applicable

- Movement: single-joint

- Performed: both legs simultaneously

Trainer/Participant Position

The participant begins by lying flat on his or her back on the floor. The participant rotates the knees upward until a 90-degree angle is formed between the legs and the floor. The participant stabilizes the legs either by grabbing the backs of the knees with the hands or by using the bar as a support. The head and back remain on the floor for the duration of the exercise.

The trainer takes position by facing the participant, standing at his or her feet. Squatting down, the trainer reaches forward and places his or her hands just above the participant's ankles with an interlocking grip. The trainer must maintain this hand position in order to avoid injury to the participant's foot, knee or ankle, and to avoid disruption of the movement.

The Movement

The participant begins the movement by simply rotating the knees upward and extending the legs until they are nearly straight. During the eccentric phase the participant slowly returns to the starting position, resisting the trainer. The participant should try to extend through a complete range of motion but only as far as they can while keeping his or her back flat to the ground. The movement is repeated until exhaustion.

The trainer provides resistance by allowing the leg extension of the participant to carry his or her body up to a standing position. During the eccentric phase the trainer provides resistance by lowering back into the squatting position. This causes gravity and the trainer's body weight to provide the majority of the resistance for the participant and allows for a smoother movement of the exercise.

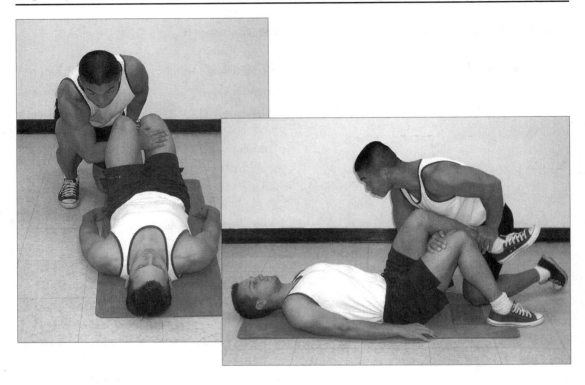

Fig. 5.4. Single leg extension.
Above: starting position.
Below: finishing position.

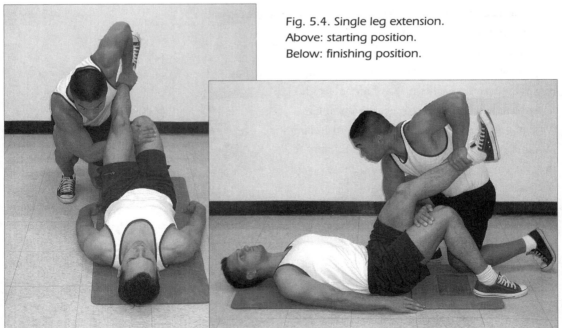

Single Leg Extension

Introduction

■ Primary muscle: quadriceps (front of the upper leg)

■ Secondary muscle: not applicable

■ Movement: single-joint

■ Performed: one leg at a time

Trainer/Participant Position

The participant begins by lying flat on his or her back, on the floor. The knees are bent at a 45-degree angle, with the feet placed flat on the floor. The arms are placed at the sides with the palms flat against the floor for stability. The head and back remain on the floor for the duration of the exercise.

The trainer takes position by kneeling at the side of the participant, facing them. The trainer lifts one leg of the participant, and using the opposite arm, loops it under the lifted leg of the participant and over the opposite leg. The trainer's hand rests slightly above the participant's stable leg. The trainer's opposite hand is positioned just above the ankle with a flat palm on the leg to be extended by the participant. This position creates support for the participant's knee as well as providing a stable platform for the trainer.

The Movement

The participant begins the movement by simply extending the leg upward until it is nearly straight. During the eccentric phase, the participant slowly returns to the starting position, resisting the trainer. The participant should try to extend through a complete range of motion but only as far as they can without locking the knee in a completely straight position. The movement is completed when the participant can no longer extend the leg.

The trainer provides resistance by allowing the participant to push the trainer's arm upward in an arcing motion. During the eccentric phase, the trainer pushes downward, using the chest, shoulder and arm. The trainer has created a position of leverage, kneeling on the knee furthest from the participant. Because the axis of the trainer's shoulder is higher than that of the participant's knee, the trainer can provide resistance fairly easily, using the arm, shoulder, and chest. The trainer should be conscious to keep an open palm above the participant's ankle to create a smooth motion for the movement.

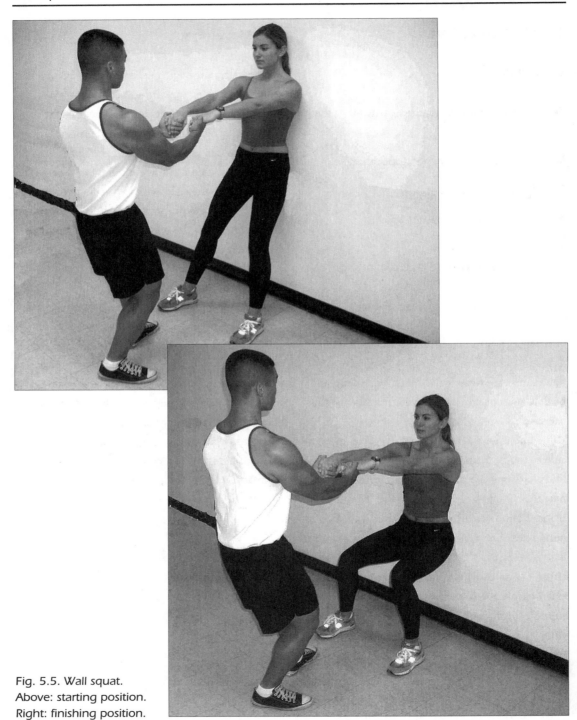

Fig. 5.5. Wall squat.
Above: starting position.
Right: finishing position.

Wall Squat

Introduction

- Primary muscle: quadriceps (front of the upper leg)

- Secondary muscle: not applicable

- Movement: isometric

- Performed: one motion

Trainer/Participant Position

The participant begins by standing with his or her back flat against a wall. The participant then positions his or her feet far enough from the wall that the legs form a 90-degree angle when the participant slides down the wall into a "sitting" position. It may take a few times of repositioning to find the proper distance. It is important to find the proper foot positioning in order to avoid knee strain and potential injury. The back and head remain flat against the wall for the duration of the exercise.

The trainer takes position by directly facing the participant, within arms reach. The primary responsibility of the trainer during the wall squat is to act as a spotter, making sure that the participant maintains proper positioning and does not fall. The trainer's arms remain extended toward the participant as a spotting technique.

The Movement

From a standing position the participant slides down the wall into a sitting position, maintaining a 90-degree angle with the legs. From the side it should appear as if the participant is sitting in an invisible chair. The participant does not move during the exercise, maintaining the position for as long as possible. The participant should keep his or her back, shoulders, and head against the wall throughout the duration of the exercise, helping to maintain constant pressure on the quadriceps. The participant's arms should be extended ready to grab the arms of the trainer as muscle fatigue approaches. The participant maintains the "sitting" position as long as possible.

The trainer, standing directly in front of the participant, should have his or her arms extended, ready to pull the participant up to the standing position. The trainer must make sure a 90-degree angle is maintained during the exercise, and be aware of the participant's fatigue level, avoiding injury from improper positioning or a fall.

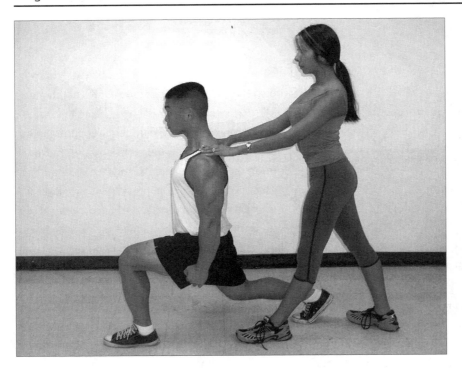

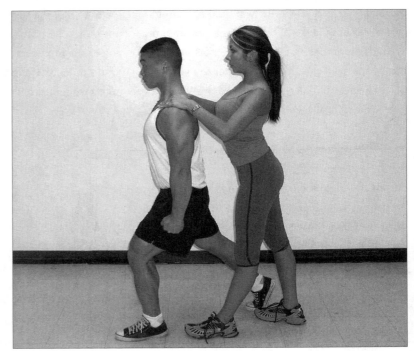

Fig. 5.6. Lunges.
Above: starting position.
Right: finishing position.

Lunges

Introduction

- Primary muscle: quadriceps (front of the upper leg)

- Secondary muscles: hamstring (back of the upper leg), glutes (buttocks) and calves

- Movement: multi-joint

- Performed: one leg at a time

Trainer/Participant Position

From an upright and standing position with the feet shoulder-width apart, the participant steps forward with one leg. After taking the initial step, the participant bends the knee until a 90-degree angle is formed with the leg. It is important to achieve a 90-degree angle in order to avoid injury to the knee and to maximize the effectiveness of the exercise. The participant maintains an upright position with the back straight, chest out, and chin up throughout the duration of the exercise.

The trainer takes position directly behind the participant with the hands placed on the participant's shoulders. The trainer's feet are placed shoulder-width apart in an offset stance. The trainer should maintain a firm grip but must be careful not to clench the participant's shoulders too tightly.

The Movement

With the participant in the starting position (leg forming a 90-degree angle) the participant pushes upward, straightening the lead leg, squeezing the quadriceps. During the eccentric phase, the participant slowly returns to the starting position, resisting the trainer, who is applying constant downward pressure. The movement is completed after fatigue is reached in one leg.

The trainer applies resistance by leaning downward, forcing his or her own weight onto the participant's body. This is consistent during each phase of the exercise. The trainer acts as a force multiplier during this exercise, causing the participant to carry the body weight of both individuals. Standing more closely to the participant, the trainer can increase resistance. The trainer, supporting more of his or her own body weight or stepping away from the participant, can decrease resistance. The trainer should be sure to apply pressure only at a direct downward angle, not pushing the participant back or forward, which can cause a loss of balance and a break in the movement.

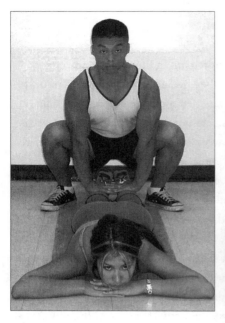

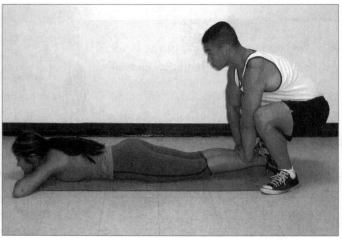

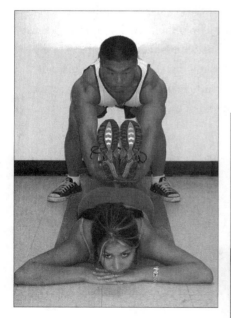

Fig. 5.7. Hamstring curl.
Above: starting position.
Below: finishing position

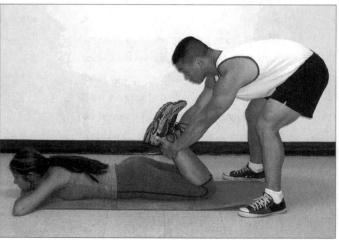

Hamstring Curl

Introduction

- Primary muscle: hamstrings (backs of the upper legs)

- Secondary muscles: glutes (buttocks), calves

- Movement: single-joint

- Performed: Simultaneously with both legs

Trainer/Participant Position

The participant begins the exercise by lying face down on the floor. The hands are placed under the chin or in the most comfortable position for the participant. The participant's legs and feet are placed together and remain that way for the duration of the exercise.

The trainer begins by standing directly over the participant's legs, approximately halfway between the ankles and the knees. This position provides the trainer with the maximum amount of leverage during the exercise, decreasing the amount of physical work needed to provide proper resistance. The trainer then assumes a squatting position with fingers interlocked. The hands are placed a few inches above the participant's ankles. This avoids unnecessary torque on the participant's knees and produces a smooth movement during the exercise.

The Movement

Beginning the movement by lying face down on the floor, the participant curls his or her legs slightly past a 90-degree angle, squeezing the hamstrings. During the eccentric phase the participant resists the trainer slowly back to the starting position. The movement is completed when the participant can no longer curl the legs past 90 degrees. It is important for the participant to keep his or her hips on the ground at all times to ensure that the hamstrings are isolated.

The trainer, starting in a squatting position, provides resistance by letting the participant pull the trainer's body into a standing position. During the eccentric motion the trainer sits back down into a squatting stance, pulling the participant's legs down at the same time. The trainer gains leverage by positioning his or her body over the lever arm (over the participant's feet) at the furthest point from the rotation. This allows the trainer's body weight and gravity to do most of the work for the trainer.

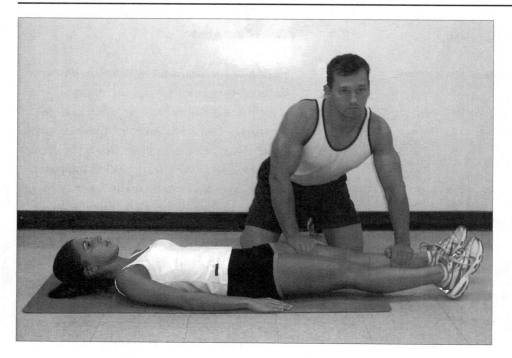

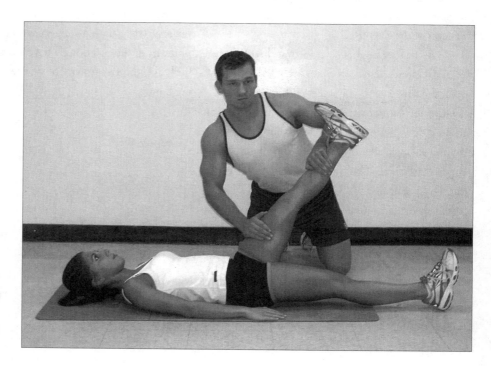

Fig. 5.8. Lying leg raise. Above: starting position. Right: finishing position.

Lying Leg Raise

Introduction

- ■　Primary muscle: hip flexor (hip girdle)

- ■　Secondary muscle: quadriceps (front of the upper leg)

- ■　Movement: single-joint

- ■　Performed: one leg at a time

Trainer/Participant Position

The participant begins the exercise by lying flat on his or her back on the floor. The arms are placed at the sides with the palms of the hands flat against the floor. The participant's legs are set slightly apart and remain that way for the duration of the exercise.

The trainer begins by kneeling at one side of the participant, next to the legs. The trainer selects a leg and places one hand just above the knee (on the thigh) and the other slightly above the ankle. The trainer's hands should be placed firmly at these points with the palms flat against the leg.

The Movement

Keeping the leg straight, the participant rotates the leg upward at the hip, raising the leg off of the floor. The participant should rotate the leg upward as high as possible in order to achieve a full range of motion. The participant then resists the movement back to the starting position and repeats the exercise. It is important for the participant to keep the leg straight throughout the duration of the exercise. Any bend in the knee will cause a break in the movement, and a loss of isolation.

The trainer, kneeling beside the participant, provides resistance by pushing against the upward movement of the leg. During the eccentric motion the trainer pushes the participant's leg downward toward the floor. The small range of motion and the trainer's position above the participant's leg provides a dramatic leverage advantage for the trainer.

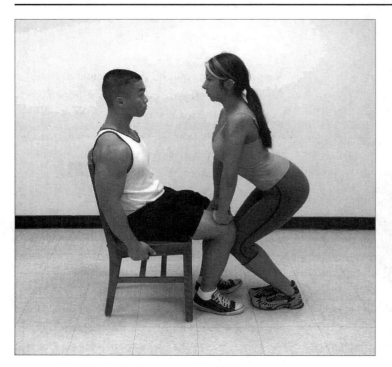

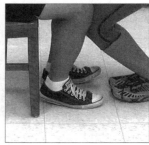

Fig. 5.9. Seated calf raise.
Above: starting position and
detail.
Right and below: finishing
position and detail.

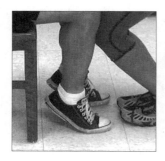

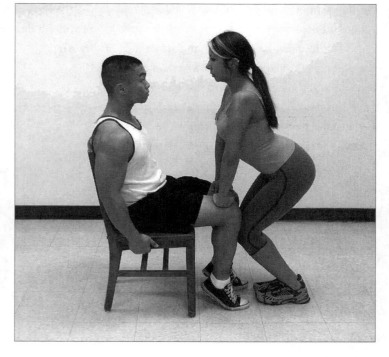

Seated Calf Raise

Introduction

- Primary muscle: gastrocnemius (calves)

- Secondary Muscle: not applicable

- Movement: multi-joint

- Performed: simultaneously with both legs

Trainer/Participant Position

The participant begins the exercise by sitting in a sturdy chair with his or her back firmly against the back of the chair. The feet, placed flat on the floor, can be positioned from a few inches apart to shoulder-width apart.

The trainer takes position by standing directly in front of the participant. Leaning over, the trainer places the palm of each hand just above the participant's knees, at the lower thigh. The trainer should then lean over, so that his or her chest is directly above the participant's knees. The trainer's arms remain straight and perpendicular to the floor, creating leverage.

The Movement

The participant begins the movement by raising his or her heels off of the ground as high as possible, while the toes remain stationary and firmly on the ground. During the eccentric phase the participant slowly returns to the starting position, resisting against the body weight of the trainer. The exercise is completed when the participant can no longer raise his or her heels from the ground.

The trainer provides resistance by keeping his or her arms straight and allowing the participant to push the body slightly upward. The trainer gains leverage by positioning his or her chest above the point of rotation (the participant's knees). The trainer's body weight and the ability to stay above the participant's knees largely provide resistance during the exercise.

6.

Exercises for the Chest

The chest is one of the largest muscle groups in the upper body. It consists of the pectoralis major (sternum and clavicular), pectoralis minor, and serratus anterior. Due to the triangular pattern of the muscle fiber, the chest has tremendous strength. It is the muscle group from which all "pushing" exercises of the body originate.

The exercises contained in this chapter are the following:

- Bench Press

- Incline Bench Press

- Dumbbell Bench Press

- Dumbbell Incline Press

- Resisted Push Up

- Standing Push Up

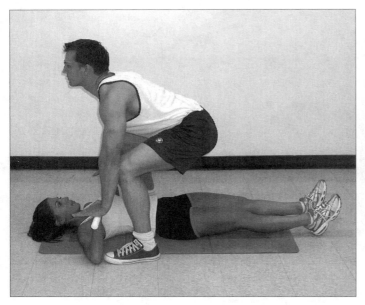

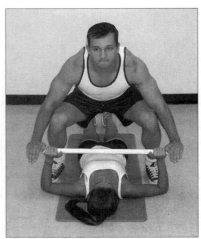

Fig. 6.1. Bench press.
Top: starting position.
Bottom: finishing position.

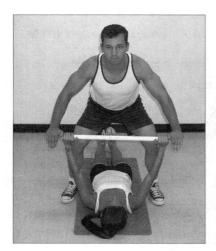

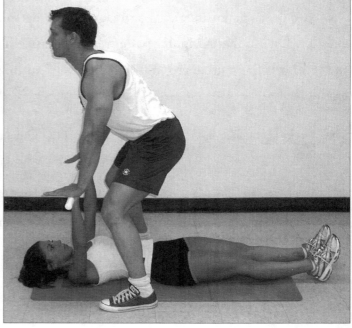

Bench Press

Introduction

- Primary muscles: pectoralis major and minor (overall chest)

- Secondary muscles: triceps (back of the upper arm) and anterior deltoid (front of the shoulder)

- Movement: multi-joint

- Performed: simultaneous arm movement

Trainer/Participant Position

The participant begins the exercise by lying flat on his or her back. The legs are positioned together, flat on the floor. The participant should position the hands on the bar shoulder-width apart, and take a firm but not tight overhand grip. Starting position for the exercise will be with the participant's arms in a perpendicular plane to the rest of the body, with the triceps in a straight line with the shoulders. The triceps should be resting on the ground.

The trainer takes position by standing directly over the participant's abdomen. Squatting down, the trainer places his or her hands directly outside the participant's hands on the bar. The grip should be firm but light, to create a smooth motion during the exercise. The trainer's arms should be straight and in a vertical plane, perpendicular to the floor. The trainer's chest should be directly over the bar in order to create leverage.

The Movement

Beginning the exercise in the starting position, the participant presses straight upward with a vertical motion, squeezing the chest during the movement. The arms extend to a nearly straight position without locking out the elbows. During the eccentric phase, the participant slowly returns to the starting position. The movement is completed when the participant can no longer extend his or her arms.

The trainer provides resistance by allowing his or her body to be pushed from a squatting position into a more upright position during the concentric phase of the movement. During the eccentric phase, the trainer returns to a squatting position, pushing the bar downward. By keeping the arms in a vertical plane and the chest over the bar, the trainer's body weight and gravity provide most of the resistance during the exercise.

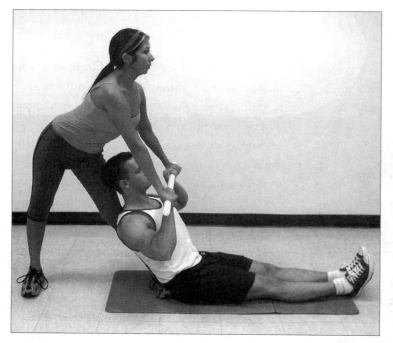

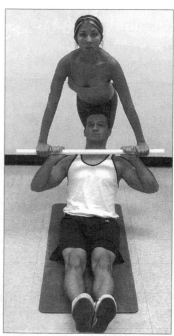

Fig. 6.2. Incline bench press. Above: starting position. Below: finishing position.

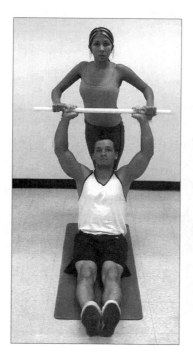

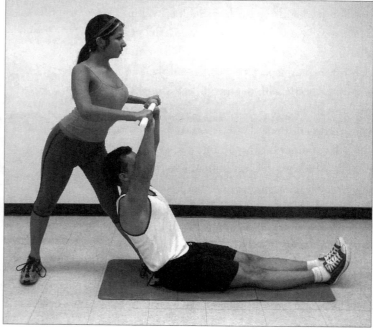

Incline Bench Press

Introduction

- Primary muscle: pectoralis minor (upper chest)

- Secondary muscles: pectoralis major (overall chest), triceps (back of the upper arm), and anterior deltoid (front of the shoulder)

- Movement: multi-joint

- Performed: simultaneously with both arms

Trainer/Participant Position

(See Setup, pages 34 and 35.) The participant begins by sitting on the floor, keeping a straight back and upright posture. The trainer takes position behind the participant in a perpendicular fashion so that the side of the trainer's foot and leg are flat against the center of the participant's back, providing support. With the alternate leg, the trainer steps out, creating a wide stance, allowing the participant to lean back. This forms a 45-degree angle from the participant's waist to the shoulders.

In this position, the participant takes a shoulder-width grip on the bar, which is placed at the clavicle. Twisting at the waist to face the same direction as the participant, the trainer leans over and positions his or her hands directly outside the participant's hands, with an open palm grip. The trainer's chest should be directly over the bar for leverage.

The Movement

At the starting position, with the bar at the participant's clavicle, the participant pushes upward in a vertical motion toward the ceiling, against the resistance of the trainer. The arms are fully extended without locking the elbows. During the eccentric phase the participant returns to the starting position, slowly resisting the trainer.

The trainer provides resistance by allowing the participant to push the trainer's body from a leaning position into a standing position. During the eccentric phase the trainer leans over, pushing the bar downward to the participant's clavicle. Leverage is gained as the trainer's chest is over the bar. While the participant's form is fairly easy to monitor in this fixed position, it is the trainer that must be aware of his or her own position. The trainer should easily be able to support the weight of the participant, but leaning too far back may cause injury to the knee of the trainer. The trainer's knee should be kept at a slight bend throughout the duration of the exercise.

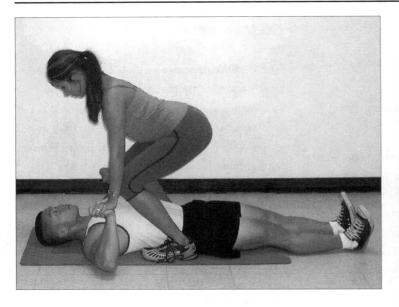

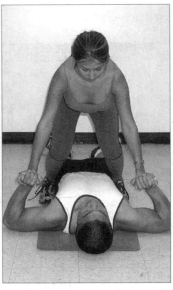

Fig. 6.3. Dumbbell bench press.
Top: starting position.
Bottom: finishing position.

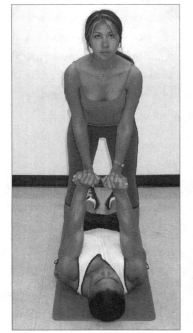

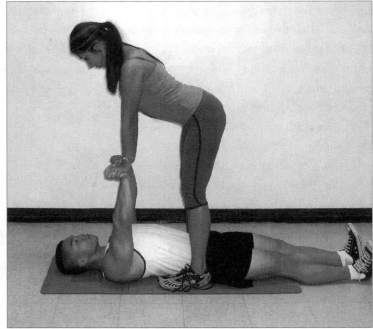

Dumbbell Bench Press

Introduction

- Primary muscle: pectoralis minor (upper chest)

- Secondary muscles: pectoralis major (overall chest), triceps (back of the upper arm), and anterior deltoid (front of the shoulder)

- Movement: multi-joint

- Performed: simultaneously with both arms

Trainer/Participant Position

The participant begins the exercise by lying flat on his or her back. The legs are positioned together, flat on the floor. The participant then rotates the arms outward from the sides of the body so that they are in the same plane as the shoulders. Rotating upward at the elbows, the upper arm is now perpendicular to the floor. Starting position for the exercise will be with the participant's arms in a perpendicular plane to the rest of the body, with the triceps in a straight line with the shoulders. The triceps should be resting on the ground.

The trainer takes a position by standing over the participant at the abdomen. Squatting down and with an open grip, the trainer takes hold of the participant's hands so that the palms meet. The trainer's arms should be straight and in a vertical plane, perpendicular to the floor. The trainer's chest should be over the bar in order to create leverage.

The Movement

The participant begins the movement by pressing his or her arms vertically upward and squeezing the chest. The arms are fully extended without locking the elbows. The participant's hands should come together at the top of the concentric movement. During the eccentric phase the participant resists the trainer slowly and steadily back to the starting position. The movement is completed when the participant can no longer push upward from the ground, reaching fatigue.

The trainer provides resistance by keeping his or her arms straight and allowing the participant to push his or her body out of the squatting position and into a standing one. During the eccentric phase of the movement the trainer provides resistance by sitting back down into a squatting position, pressing downward. By keeping the arms straight and in a vertical plane with the chest over the participant's hands, the trainer's body weight and gravity provide most of the resistance during the exercise.

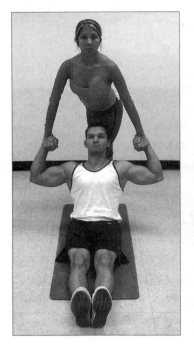
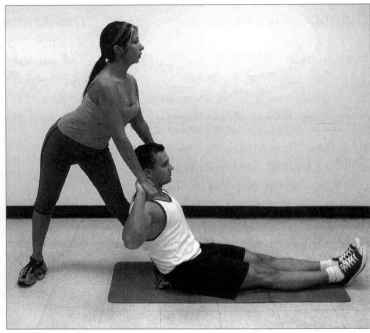

Figs. 6.4. Dumbbell incline press. Above: starting position. Below: finishing position.

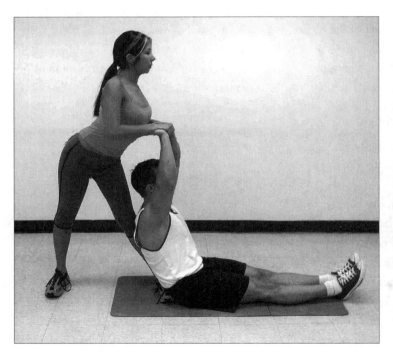
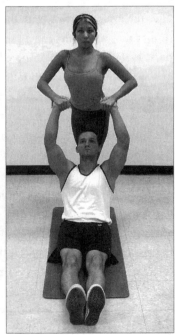

Dumbbell Incline Press

Introduction

■ Primary muscles: pectoralis minor (upper chest)

■ Secondary muscles: pectoralis major (overall chest), triceps (back of the upper arm), and anterior deltoid (front of the shoulder)

■ Movement: multi-joint

■ Performed: simultaneous movement of both arms

Trainer/Participant Position

(See Setup, pages 32 and 33.) The participant begins by sitting on the floor, keeping a straight back and upright posture. The trainer takes position behind the participant in a perpendicular fashion so that the side of the trainer's foot and leg are flat against the center of the participant's back, providing support. With the alternate leg, the trainer steps out, creating a wide stance, allowing the participant to lean back. This forms a 45-degree angle from the participant's waist to the shoulders.

In this position, the participant reaches up and takes a firm grip on the trainer's hands. Twisting at the waist, the trainer leans over the participant and grasps the participant's hands, with an open palm grip.

The Movement

At the starting position, with the hands positioned at the front of the participant's shoulders, the participant pushes upward in a vertical motion toward the ceiling, bringing the hands together at the top of the movement, against the resistance of the trainer. During the eccentric phase the trainer slowly returns to the starting position, resisting the trainer. The movement is completed when the chest is completely fatigued.

The trainer provides resistance by allowing the participant to push them up from a leaning position to a standing one. During the eccentric phase the trainer leans forward pressing the arms down. The trainer should be sure to give equal pressure from both arms to maintain participant balance and a steady movement. While the participant's form is fairly easy to monitor in this fixed position, it is the trainer that must be aware of his or her own position. The trainer should easily be able to support the weight of the participant, but leaning too far back may cause injury to the knee of the trainer. The trainer's knee should be kept at a slight bend throughout the duration of the exercise.

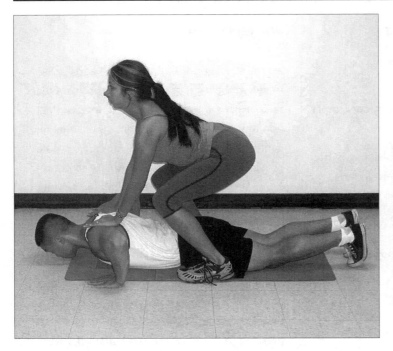
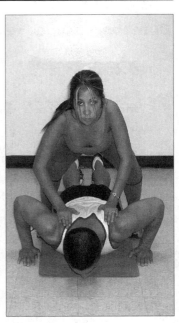

Figs. 6.5. Resisted push-ups. Above: starting position. Below: finishing position.

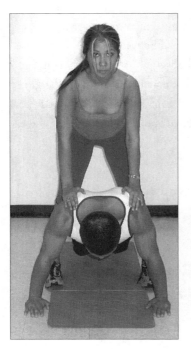
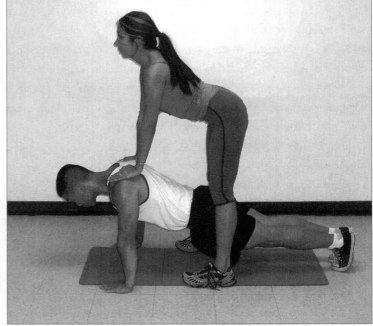

Resisted Push-Up

Introduction

- Primary muscle: pectoralis major and minor (overall chest)

- Secondary muscle: triceps (back of the upper arm)

- Movement: multi-joint

- Performed: simultaneously with both arms

Trainer/Participant Position

The participant begins by taking the standard starting position of a traditional push-up. The arms should be shoulder-width apart, on the same plane as the shoulders. The participant's feet are positioned together and the body rests on the ground.

The trainer takes position by squatting over the participant's mid-back. The trainer's hands are placed directly on or slightly below the participant's shoulder blades. The arms should be straight and perpendicular to the floor. The trainer's chest should be positioned over the mid-back to create leverage.

The Movement

The participant begins the exercise in the starting (down) position, with the arms parallel to the floor, forming a 90-degree angle. A standard push-up is performed, with the participant extending his or her arms fully, without locking the elbows. During the eccentric phase, the participant slowly returns to the starting position, resisting the trainer. The movement is completed when the participant can no longer rise from the starting position.

The trainer provides resistance by allowing the participant to push the trainer's body out of a squatting position and into a standing position. During the eccentric phase, the trainer returns to the squatting position, pushing downward against the back of the participant. The trainer maintains leverage by placing his or her body directly above the participant's body, acting as a force multiplier. The trainer is simply supplementing the effects of gravity, so little resistance is typically needed. The trainer should be sure the participant's back remains flat and the chest remains out, to avoid potential injury.

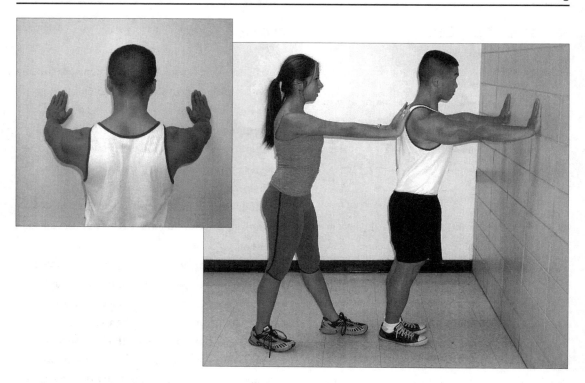

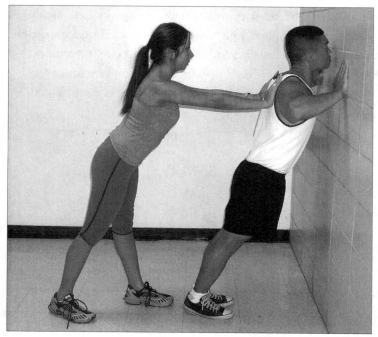

Fig. 6.6. Standing push-up.
Top left: set-up.
Above right: starting position.
Lower left: finishing position.

Standing Push-Up

Introduction

■ Primary muscles: pectoralis major and minor (overall chest)

■ Secondary muscles: triceps (back of the upper arm) and posterior deltoid (back of the shoulder)

■ Movement: multi-joint

■ Performed: simultaneously with both arms

Trainer/Participant Position

The participant begins by facing a stable wall and placing his or her hands, palms flat, against the wall. The arms should be shoulder-width apart, at shoulder height, so that they are parallel to the floor. The participant's feet are placed side by side and should be far enough from the wall that the arms are straight but the palms remain in constant contact with the wall.

The trainer takes position by standing an arm's length away from the participant. The feet are shoulder-width apart and in an offset stance. Then, the trainer extends his or her arms and leans forward to place the palms of the hands flat on the participant's shoulder blades.

The Movement

The participant begins by pressing outward from the wall. The arms are fully extended without locking the elbows. During the eccentric phase, the participant slowly returns to the starting position, resisting the trainer. The movement is repeated until the triceps reach complete exhaustion.

The trainer provides resistance by leaning forward, allowing the participant to push the trainer's body back. During the eccentric phase, the trainer leans forward, taking a step if necessary and pushing with the arms. The trainer maintains leverage by leaning his or her body forward, causing the participant to absorb the weight. As the participant's arms are extended, the participant significantly reduces the trainer's mechanical advantage. But as the participant gets closer to the wall, they will lose that mechanical advantage and the movement will become increasingly difficult.

7.

Exercises for the Back

For the purposes of this book, the back consists of the erector spinae, mid-rhomboids, latimus dorsi, and the trapezius. Although some of the muscles listed are technically associated with the shoulder, they also play a significant role in most exercises of the back. Unlike many muscle groups, the muscles of the back serve a variety of different functions. The erector spinae is primarily responsible for the movement and bending of the spine, while the rhomboids and latimus dorsi give width and density to the posterior musculature. Most "pulling" exercises originate from the back.)

Here is a list of the exercises contained in this chapter:

- One-Arm Lateral Adductor

- One-Arm Lateral Pull

- Seated Row

- Bent-Over Row

- Pull-Up

- Superman

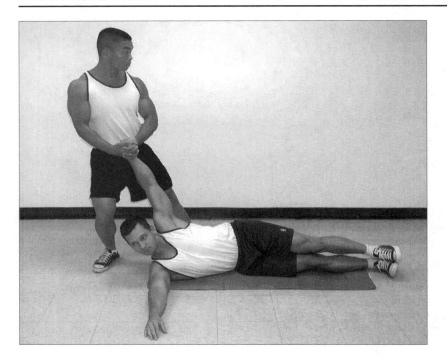

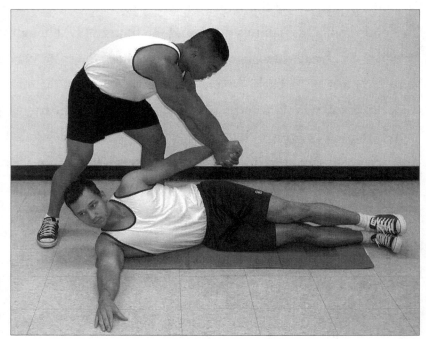

Fig. 7.1. One-arm lateral
adductor.
Above: starting position.
Right: finishing position.

One-Arm Lateral Adductor

Introduction

- Primary muscle: latimus dorsi (side of the back)

- Secondary muscles: biceps (front of the upper arm), forearm

- Movement: single-joint

- Performed: one side at a time

Trainer/Participant Position

The participant begins by lying on the floor on his or her side. The arm against the floor is extended perpendicular to the body to create a base of support. After the base of support is created, the participant extends the top arm upward toward the ceiling.

The trainer takes position directly behind the participant, standing at the head and shoulders. Using an interlocking grip, the trainer firmly grasps the participant's extended hand and rotates the arm into the starting position, slightly past 90 degrees. Finally, the trainer should be aligned in the same direction as the participant's body (toward the participant's feet).

The Movement

The participant begins the exercise by rotating the arm downward, to the side of the body. To complete the movement, the participant allows the trainer to pull his or her arm slowly back to the starting position. The arm must remain straight throughout the duration of the exercise in order to isolate the latimus dorsi (side of the back). Any bend at the elbow will cause a break in the movement.

The trainer provides resistance by allowing the participant to pull them forward as the arm is rotated down to the side. The trainer will have to step forward and lean down as the participant completes the concentric phase. During the eccentric phase, the trainer steps back to the original position, slowly rotating the participant's arm back to the starting point.

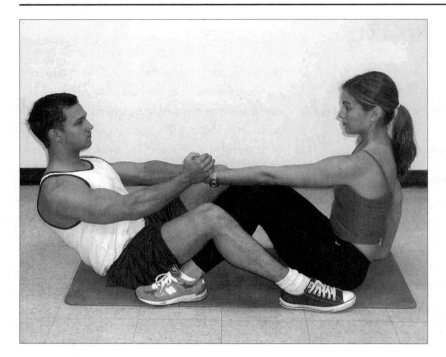

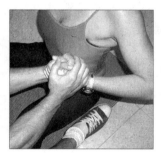

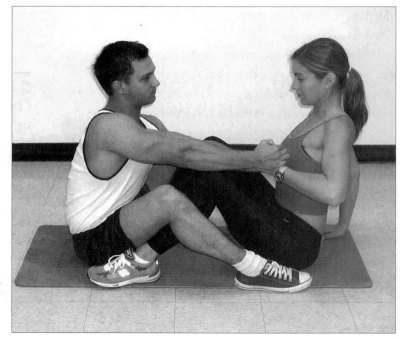

Fig. 7.2. One-arm lateral pull.
Top: starting position.
Above: hand position detail.
Right: finishing position.

One-Arm Lateral Pull

Introduction

- Primary muscle: latimus dorsi (side of the back)

- Secondary muscles: biceps (front of the upper arm), forearm

- Movement: multi-joint

- Performed: one side at a time

Trainer/Participant Position

The participant begins by sitting on the floor with the knees bent at a 45-degree angle. The feet are placed firmly on the floor shoulder-width apart forming a solid base. The participant places one hand on the floor for support as the opposite arm is extended forward so that it is parallel to the ground. The back remains straight and the chest out for the duration of the exercise.

The trainer assumes a seated position directly facing the participant. The trainer then moves forward and interlocks legs with the participant for support, with the trainer's legs on the outside. The trainer's feet are placed on the floor directly outside the participant's hips and the trainer's knees are directly outside the participant's knees (or at the appropriate distance based on the height of the trainer and participant). The trainer grasps the participant's extended hand with one hand and holds onto the participant's wrist with the other to provide support.

The Movement

The participant, whose upper body remains facing the trainer in a fixed position throughout the exercise, pulls the arm around the side of the body in an arcing motion. This motion continues until the elbow moves past the plane of the back. The arm should remain parallel to the floor throughout the duration of the exercise. The movement is completed as the participant resists the trainer through the eccentric phase of the exercise, back to the starting position. The exercise is completed when the participant reaches fatigue.

The trainer provides resistance by allowing the participant to pull the trainer's body forward during the concentric motion. During the eccentric motion, the trainer leans the upper body backward, pulling the participant's arm back to the starting point. The trainer's function is to provide a counterbalance to the participant, simultaneously providing support and resistance.

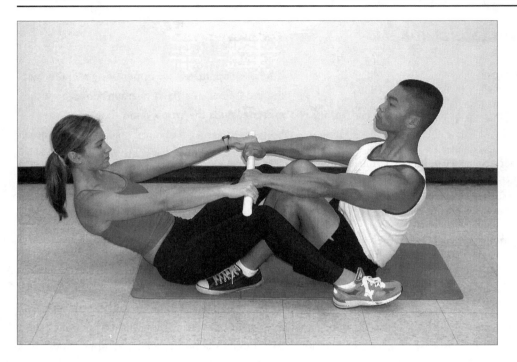

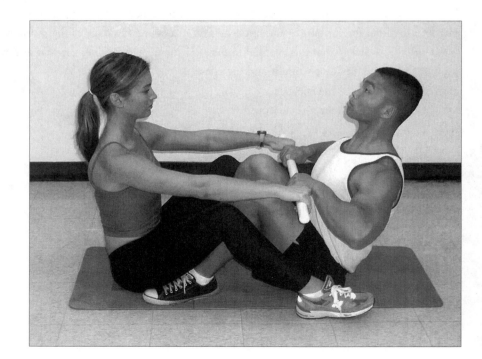

Fig. 7.3. Seated
row.
Above: starting
position.
Right: finishing
position.

76

Seated Row

Introduction

- Primary muscle: mid-rhomboids (middle of the back)

- Secondary muscle: latimus dorsi (sides of the back)

- Movement: multi-joint

- Performed: simultaneously with both arms

Trainer/Participant Position

The participant begins by sitting on the floor with the knees bent at a 45-degree angle. The feet are placed firmly on the floor shoulder-width apart forming a solid base. The participant then grasps the bar with an overhand grip, making sure the hands are shoulder-width apart. The participant's back remains straight and the chest remains out for the duration of the exercise.

The trainer assumes a seated position directly facing the participant. The trainer then moves forward and interlocks legs with the participant for support, with the trainer's legs on the outside. The trainer's feet are placed at on the floor directly outside the participant's hips and the trainer's knees are outside the participant's knees (depending on the height of the participant and trainer). The trainer then grasps the bar directly outside the hands of the participant with a firm grip.

The Movement

The participant begins the exercise by leaning back slightly at the hips, keeping the back straight and the chest out. The participant pulls the bar into the lower chest, keeping the arms parallel to the floor and the elbows out. This helps to isolate the mid-back region. During the eccentric phase, the participant slowly returns to the starting position, resisting the trainer. The movement is complete when the participant reaches fatigue. Keeping the arms straight, the trainer allows the participant to pull his or her body forward at the hips during the concentric phase. During the eccentric phase, the trainer leans back, pulling the participant's arms back to the starting point.

The trainer functions primarily as a counterbalance to provide resistance, leaning the body backward at the hips to provide adequate resistance. The trainer should make sure the participant's upper body remains stationary and does not move forward or back at the hips.

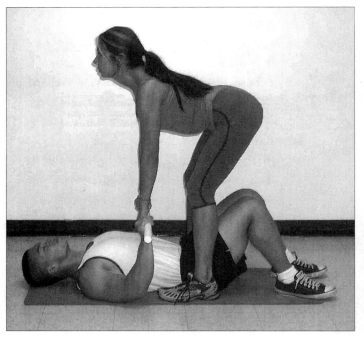
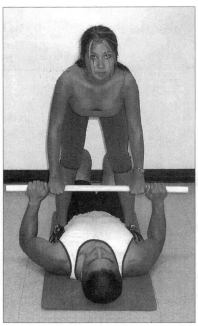

Fig. 7.4. Bent-over row.
Top: starting position.
Bottom: finishing position.

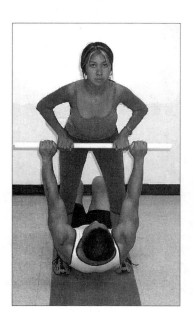
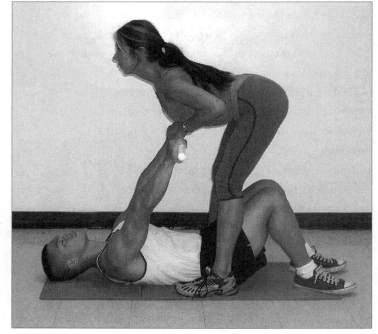

Bent-Over Row

Introduction

- Primary muscles: latimus dorsi (sides of the back) and mid-rhomboids (middle of the back)

- Secondary muscles: biceps (front of the upper arm) and forearms

- Movement: multi-joint

- Performed: simultaneous arm movement

Trainer/Participant Position

The trainer takes position first during this exercise by lying flat on his or her back on the floor. The trainer then takes a wide, overhand grip on the bar at chest level. The grip should be firm, but loose enough to maintain stability during the exercise.

The participant stands over the trainer, approximately at the abdomen, bending slightly at the knees. The participant then leans over at the waist, so that the back is nearly parallel to the floor. The participant then reaches down and grasps the bar directly inside the hands of the trainer using an overhand grip. The participant should maintain a posture with a straight back, chest out, and chin up throughout the duration of the exercise.

The Movement

The participant begins the movement by pulling the bar in a vertical motion toward the lower chest. During the concentric motion the participant should attempt to relax the arms as much as possible and concentrate on squeezing the shoulder blades together. Although it will be impossible to make the shoulder blades meet, it will help the participant to isolate the muscles in the mid-back. During the eccentric phase, the participant slowly lowers the bar to the starting position. Because of the positioning, the trainer must rely primarily on the strength of his or her arms to provide the necessary resistance. During the concentric phase the trainer resists against the participant as they pull the bar upward to the lower chest. During the eccentric phase the trainer slowly pulls the bar back down to the starting position.

The trainer needs to pay close attention to the participant's form, making sure the chest remains out and the back stays flat. To avoid injury, the participant's back should never be bent.

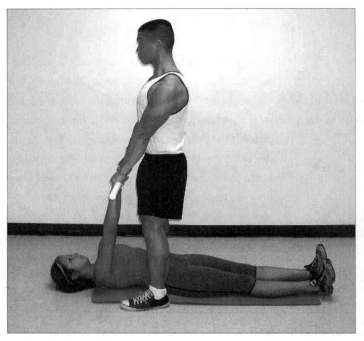

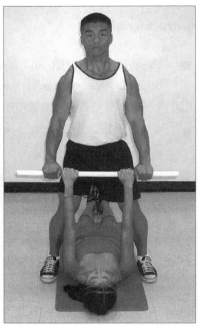

Fig. 7.4. Pull-up.
Top: starting position.
Bottom: finishing position.

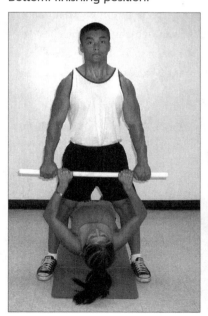

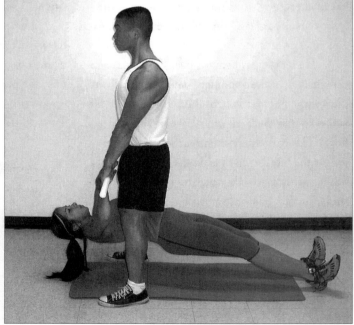

Pull-Up

Introduction

- Primary muscles: latimus dorsi (sides of the back), and mid-rhomboids (middle of the back)

- Secondary muscles: biceps (front of the upper arms), and forearms

- Movement: multi-joint

- Performed: one motion

Trainer/Participant Position

The participant assumes a starting position by lying flat on his or her back on the floor. The participant's feet and legs are placed together and remain in this position throughout the duration of the exercise.

After the participant assumes position on the floor, the trainer takes position by standing directly over the participant's waist. The feet should be positioned in a wide stance to form a stable base for the exercise. The trainer then takes a wide overhand grip on the bar. The participant then reaches up and takes an overhand grip on the bar, just inside the trainer's hands. The participant's arms should be perpendicular to the floor, with the hands positioned shoulder-width apart.

The Movement

Keeping the body rigid with a straight back and chest out, the participant pulls his or her body up to the bar, at the chest. As the body is pulled up, only the heels remain on the floor. During the eccentric phase of the movement, the participant slowly lowers the body towards the floor, stopping a few inches from the ground. The movement is completed when the participant can no longer pull the body upward.

The trainer functions primarily as a spotter, supporting the weight of the participant with the bar. This causes gravity (on the participant's own body) to provide resistance during the exercise.

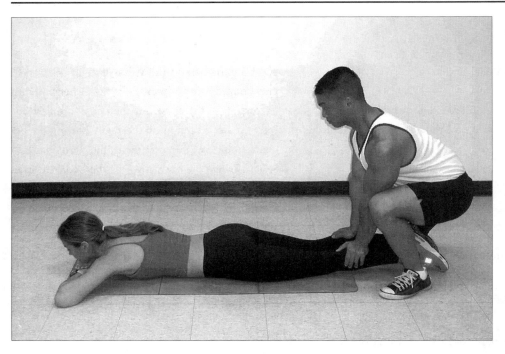

Fig. 7.4. Superman. Above: starting position. Below: finishing position.

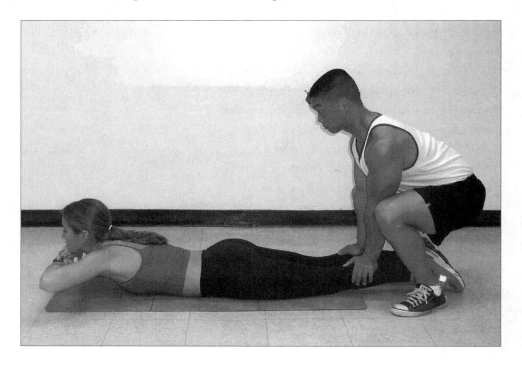

Superman

Introduction

- Primary muscle: lower back

- Secondary muscle: glutes (buttocks), and abdominals

- Movement: single-joint

- Performed: one motion

Trainer/Participant Position

The participant begins by lying face down on the floor. The hands are then placed under the chin, where they remain for the duration of the exercise. The knees and ankles are brought together to provide a base for the exercise.

The trainer takes position directly behind the participant's feet. Kneeling down, the trainer grasps the participant's legs just above the ankles. The trainer's chest should be above the participant's feet, so that the trainer's weight holds the participant's lower body firmly down during the exercise.

The Movement

Beginning the movement with the body flat against the ground, the participant raises his or her upper body from the waist, to its fullest extent. After a brief pause at the top of the movement, the participant returns to the starting position. The exercise is completed when the participant's lower back reaches fatigue. During the movement, the participant's hands stay firmly tucked under the chin, and the legs remain on the ground.

The trainer functions primarily as a spotter during the exercise, ensuring the participant's legs remain stable on the ground and a full range of motion is reached during the movement. The trainer maintains a leverage advantage with the weight of his or her body at the furthest point of the lever arm (the participant's feet), away from the axis of rotation.

8.

Exercises for the Shoulders

The shoulder, also referred to as the shoulder girdle, is comprised of several different muscles. Those muscles are the deltoids, rotator group, and trapezius. Additionally, the rhomboids and latimus dorsi are also part of the shoulder muscle group although they can also be associated with the back. The shoulder joint has a tremendous range of motion due to the fact that it is not a true ball and socket joint as with other joints in the body. It is really a ball and semi-socket joint. Because of this, extra care should be taken during shoulder exercises as the shoulder is easier to injure.

The exercises contained in this chapter are the following:

- Military Press

- Dumbbell Shoulder Press

- Half Arnold Shoulder Press

- Upright Row

- Side-Lateral Raise

- Front Raises

- Rear Deltoid Rotation

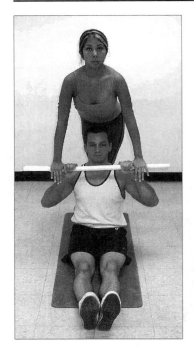
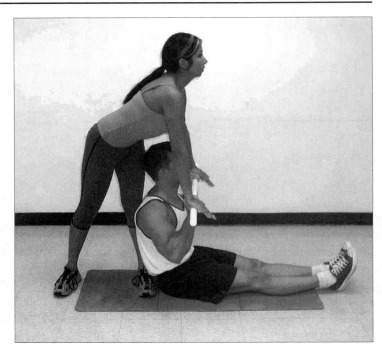

Fig. 8.1. Military press. Above: starting position. Below: finishing position.

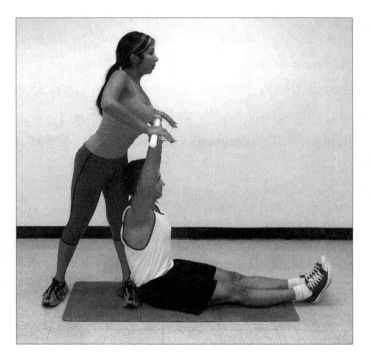
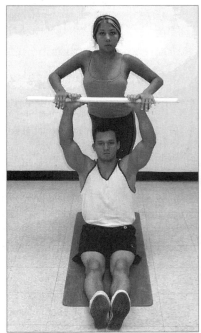

Military Press

Introduction

- Primary muscle: deltoids (all of the shoulder)

- Secondary muscle: triceps (back of the arm)

- Movement: multi-joint

- Performed: simultaneously with both arms

Trainer/Participant Position

(See Setup, pages 34–35) The participant begins by sitting on the floor, keeping a straight back and upright posture. The trainer takes position behind the participant in a perpendicular fashion so that the side of the trainer's foot and leg are flat against the center of the participant's back. With the alternate leg, the trainer steps back slightly, creating a solid base for balance and support of the participant's back. The participant should maintain a posture of a straight back with the chest out for the duration of the exercise.

In this position, the participant takes a shoulder-width grip on the bar, which is placed directly in front of the participant's nose. This causes the participant's arms to be parallel with the floor. Twisting at the waist, the trainer leans over the participant and positions his or her hands directly outside the participant's hands, with an open palm grip. The trainer's chest should be directly above the bar for leverage.

The Movement

At the starting position, with the bar at the participant's nose, the participant pushes upward in a vertical motion toward the ceiling, against the resistance of the trainer. The arms should fully extend, without locking. During the eccentric phase, the participant slowly returns to the starting position, resisting the trainer. The movement is completed when the participant can no longer press upward.

The trainer provides resistance by allowing the participant to push his or her body out of a leaning position and into a standing position. During the eccentric phase, the trainer leans over at the waist, pressing the bar downward. Leverage is gained as the trainer's center of gravity (the chest) is above the bar. While the participant's form is fairly easy to monitor in this fixed position, it is the trainer who must be aware of his or her own position. The trainer should easily be able to support the participant, but should make sure the participant maintains an upright position, not leaning forward or back. The trainer also needs to be sure he or she is giving resistance in a vertical plane (straight up and down) and not pushing the participant forward or back.

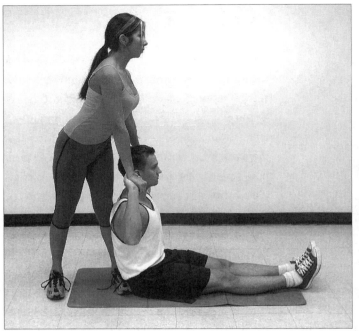
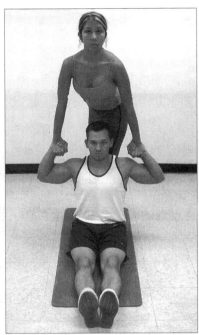

Fig. 8.2. Dumbbell shoulder press. Above: starting position. Below: finishing position.

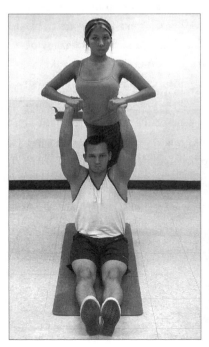
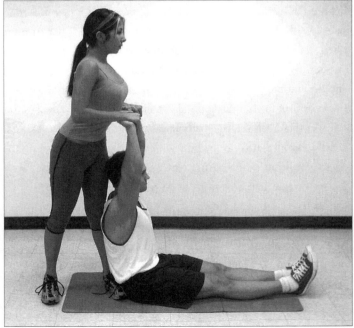

Dumbbell Shoulder Press

Introduction

- Primary muscles: overall deltoid (overall shoulder)

- Secondary muscle: triceps (back of the upper arm)

- Movement: multi-joint

- Performed: simultaneously with both arms

Trainer/Participant Position

(See Setup, pages 34–35) The participant begins by sitting on the floor, keeping a straight back and upright posture. The trainer takes position behind the participant in a perpendicular fashion so that the side of the trainer's foot and leg are flat against the center of the participant's back. With the alternate leg, the trainer steps back slightly, creating a solid base for balance and for support of the participant's back. The participant should maintain a posture of a straight back with the chest out for the duration of the exercise.

Once in the setup position, the participant reaches up until the triceps (back of the arms) are parallel to the floor. Twisting at the waist, the trainer leans over and firmly grasps the participant's hands, so that the palms of the trainer and participant are flat against one another.

The Movement

At the starting position, the participant pushes upward in a vertical motion toward the ceiling, against the resistance of the trainer. The arms are extended until they are nearly straight, without locking out the elbows. During the eccentric phase the participant slowly returns to the starting position with the triceps parallel to the ground. The movement is completed when the participant can no longer press upward.

The trainer provides resistance by allowing the participant to push the trainer's body from a leaning position to more of an upright position. During the eccentric phase, the trainer provides resistance by leaning over at the waist and pushing downward with the arms. The trainer that must be aware of his or her own position during the exercise. The trainer should easily be able to support the participant, but should make sure the participant maintains an upright position, not leaning forward or back. The trainer also needs to be sure they are providing resistance in a vertical plane (straight up and down) and not pushing the participant forward or back.

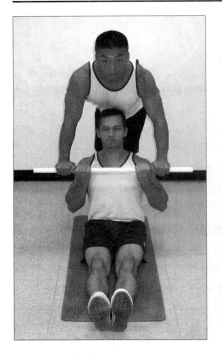
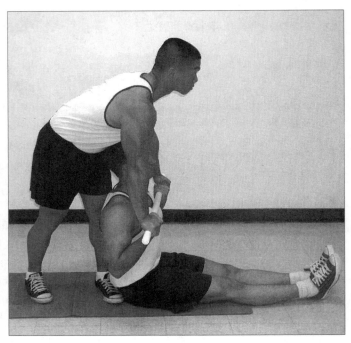

Fig. 8.3 Half Arnold shoulder press. Above: starting position. Below: finishing position.

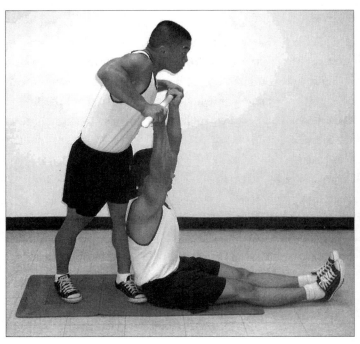
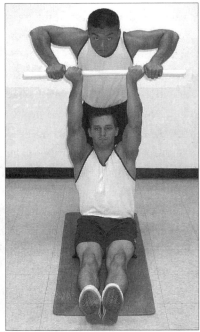

Half Arnold Shoulder Press

Introduction

- Primary muscle: anterior deltoid (front of the shoulder)

- Secondary muscle: triceps (back of the upper arm)

- Movement: multi-joint

- Performed: simultaneously with both arms

Trainer/Participant Position

(See Setup, pages 34–35.) The participant begins by sitting on the floor, keeping a straight back and upright posture. The trainer takes position behind the participant in a perpendicular fashion, so that the side of the trainer's foot and leg are flat against the center of the participant's back. With the alternate leg, the trainer steps back slightly creating a solid base for balance and for support of the participant's back. The participant should maintain a posture of a straight back with the chest out for the duration of the exercise.

In this position, the participant's elbows are at 135-degree angle and the arms are resting on top of the rib cage. The hands should grip the bar about shoulder-width apart and the palms are facing the participant. The bar should be just below the participant's chin. Twisting at the waist to face the upper body in the same direction as the participant, the trainer leans over and places his or her hands on the bar directly outside the hands of the participant. The trainer's chest should be directly above the bar for leverage.

The Movement

The participant begins by pressing upward in a vertical motion, raising the bar toward the ceiling. The arms are fully extended without locking the elbows. During the eccentric phase the bar is slowly lowered back to its original position against the resistance of the trainer. The movement is completed when the participant is no longer able to press upward.

The trainer provides resistance by allowing the participant to push the trainer's body from a leaning position to more of an upright position. During the eccentric phase, the trainer provides resistance by leaning over at the waist and pushing downward with the arms. Leverage is gained as the trainer's center of gravity remains over the bar. The trainer must be aware of his or her own position during the exercise. The trainer should easily be able to support the participant, but should make sure the participant maintains an upright position, not leaning forward or back. The trainer also needs to be sure they are providing resistance in a vertical plane (straight up and down) and not pushing the participant forward or back.

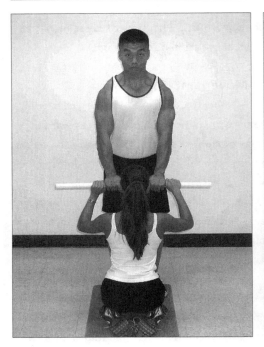
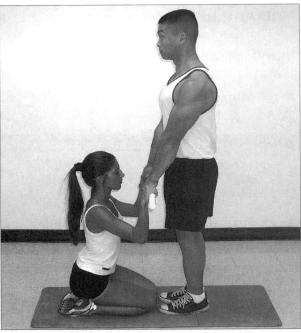

Fig. 8.4. Upright row. Above: starting position. Below: finishing position.

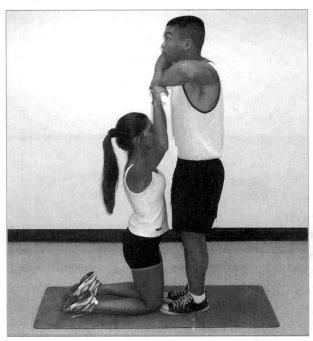
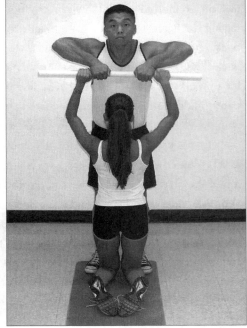

Upright Row

Introduction

■ Primary muscle: deltoids (entire shoulder)

■ Secondary muscles: trapezius (upper mid-back), and forearms

■ Movement: multi-joint

■ Performed: simultaneously with both arms

Trainer/Participant Position

The participant begins the exercise in a standing position with the feet placed shoulder-width apart and the knees slightly bent. The participant then takes an overhand grip on the bar slightly inside the width of the shoulders. The participant's back remains straight and the chest remains out for the duration of the exercise.

The trainer assumes a kneeling position directly in front of the participant, sitting on his or her own lower legs. The trainer should be positioned as close to the feet of the participant as possible in order to maximize leverage. The trainer then firmly grips the bar directly outside of the participant's hands, using an overhand grip with thumbs on the same side of the bar as the fingers.

The Movement

Beginning the exercise with the arms straight and the bar in front of the upper thighs, the participant pulls the bar upward in a vertical motion toward the chin. The participant stops the concentric movement when the upper arms become parallel to the ground. During the eccentric phase, the participant slowly returns to the starting position, resisting the trainer. The movement is completed when the participant reaches fatigue.

The trainer provides resistance by allowing the participant to pull them out of the sitting position into an upright kneeling position. During the eccentric movement, the trainer returns to a sitting position, pulling the bar downward with them. The trainer is able to provide adequate resistance by positioning his or her body close to the body of the participant and remaining as close to the bar as possible. By doing so, gravity is able to provide a significant amount of the work, as the participant has to pull the trainer's body upward.

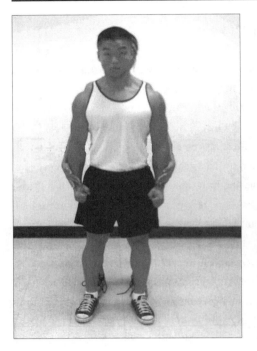
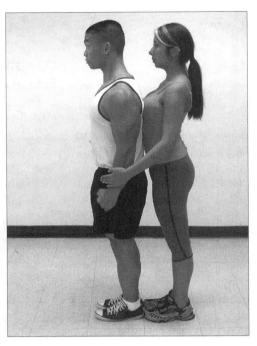

Fig. 8.4. Side-lateral raises. Above: starting position. Below: finishing position.

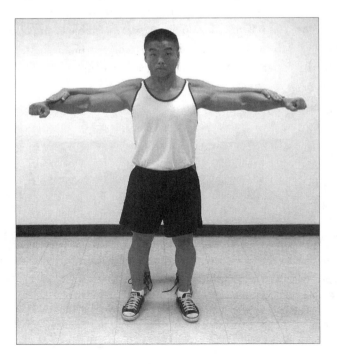
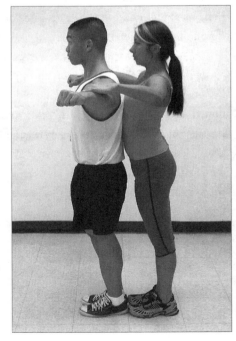

Side-Lateral Raise

Introduction

■   Primary muscle: deltoids (the entire shoulder)

■   Secondary muscles: trapezius (upper mid-back), and rotator cuff (shoulder girdle)

■   Movement: multi-joint

■   Performed: simultaneously with both arms

Trainer/Participant Position

The participant begins the exercise in a standing position with the feet placed shoulder-width apart and the knees slightly bent. The arms are placed at the sides with the hands parallel to the body. The participant's back remains straight and the chest remains out for the duration of the exercise.

The trainer takes position directly behind the participant. With open palms, the trainer places his or her hands just above the participant's wrists. The hands should remain flat against the participant's arms and not clench the wrists. Hand placement on or below the participant's wrists will cause a break in the movement and a lack of stability during the exercise.

The Movement

Beginning the exercise with the hands and arms parallel to the body, the participant raises the arms up to a 90-degree angle (parallel to the ground). During the eccentric phase, the participant slowly returns to the starting position, resisting the trainer. The movement is completed when the participant reaches fatigue. The trainer resists the participant as the arms rotate upward during the concentric movement. During the eccentric movement, the trainer presses the participant's arms back down to the sides of the body.

The trainer is able to provide adequate resistance because of the placement of the hands. By placing the hands as close to the end of the lever arm (away from the rotation point) as possible, a leverage advantage is created. Additionally, standing close to the participant's body allows the trainer to maximize the amount of resistance.

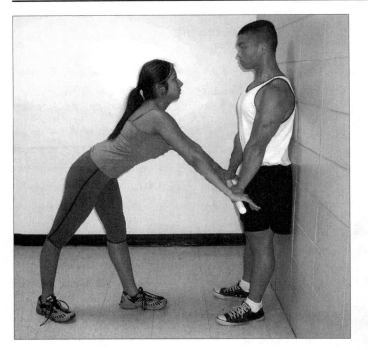

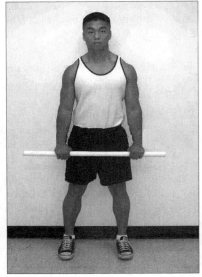

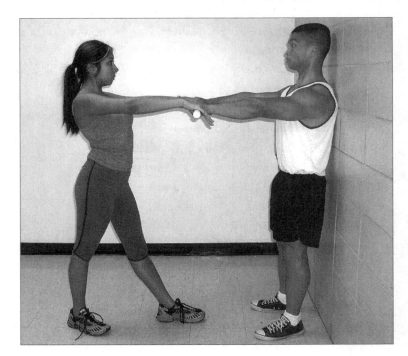

Fig. 8.5. Front raise.
Top right: setup position.
Top left: starting position.
Right: finishing position.

Front Raise

Introduction

- Primary muscle: anterior deltoids (front of the shoulder)

- Secondary muscle: not applicable

- Movement: single-joint

- Performed: simultaneously with both arms

Trainer/Participant Position

The participant begins the exercise in a standing position with his or her back flat against a wall or stable surface. The feet are positioned shoulder-width apart while keeping a slight bend to the knees. The participant uses an overhand grip on the bar, shoulder-width apart. Keeping the arms straight, the participant positions the bar across the upper thighs. The participant's hips, back, shoulders, and head remain against the wall for the duration of the exercise.

The trainer takes position in front of the participant. The trainer should stand one to two feet away from the participant in an offset stance with the feet shoulder-width apart. Bending at the waist, the trainer leans forward and grasps the bar directly outside the hands of the participant with an open palm. The grip should remain loose enough to allow the hands to roll along the bar during the movement.

The Movement

The participant begins the exercise by raising the bar in an arcing motion until the arms are parallel with the floor. After a brief pause at the top of the movement, the participant continues to resist the trainer through the eccentric phase of the movement, back to the starting position. The participant's arms remain straight for the duration of the exercise.

The trainer provides resistance by allowing the participant to push the trainer's body from a leaning position to a standing position. To be accomplished successfully, the trainer must allow the bar to rotate in the palms of his or her hands. During the eccentric phase, the trainer leans forward and pushes downward with the arms, returning to a leaning stance. The trainer maintains leverage by maintaining body weight in a position above the rotation of the arc, up to the highest point of the exercise.

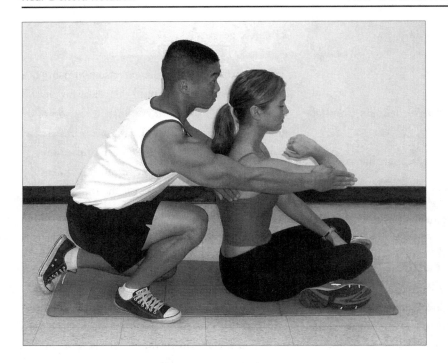

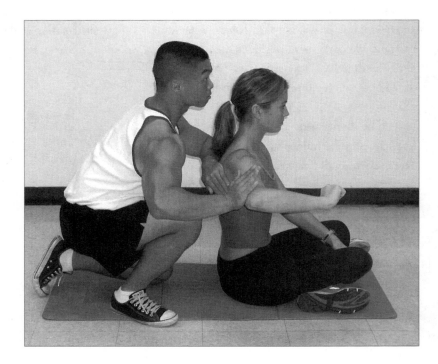

Fig. 8.6. Rear deltoid
rotation.
Above: starting position.
Right: finishing position.

Rear Deltoid Rotation

Introduction

- Primary muscle: posterior deltoids (back of the shoulder)

- Secondary muscle: rotator cuff (shoulder girdle)

- Movement: single-joint

- Performed: one arm at a time

Trainer/Participant Position

The participant begins in a seated position on the floor. The knees are bent at a 45-degree angle with the feet flat on the floor to provide a steady base. The back is straight and the chest is out in order to give the trainer a flat surface to place his or her forearm. The arm is raised until it is parallel to the floor and the elbow is bent in a 90-degree angle. The opposing arm is extended along the side of the body with the hand placed firmly on the ground to provide stability.

The trainer kneels just behind the participant with one knee on the ground while the other is placed with the foot on the ground. Then, the trainer leans forward and places his or her forearm directly across the back of the participant, at the shoulder blades. The left arm is raised until it is parallel with the participant's left upper arm. Then, the trainer places the palm of the hand on the back of the participant's elbow.

The Movement

The participant begins the movement by rotating the arm (at the shoulder joint) back toward the trainer until it forms a parallel plane to the participant's shoulders. During the eccentric movement, the participant slowly returns to the starting position, resisting the trainer. Repeat this movement, until the rear deltoid reaches complete exhaustion.

The trainer provides resistance during the exercise by pushing forward against the participant's elbow. The same holds true during the eccentric phase of the movement. Gravity plays almost no role and little leverage is needed by the trainer due to the small size and strength of the rear deltoids. Keeping this in mind, the trainer should be aware that only moderate, smooth resistance is needed to successfully complete the exercise.

99

9.

Exercises for the Triceps

The upper arm is comprised of two primary muscle groups: the biceps and the triceps. The triceps are the primary elbow extensors and are also used in shoulder extension. This chapter deals with the triceps, while Chapter 10 is devoted to the bicep group. By design, the bicep group contracts with more speed, while the triceps group is by far the stronger of the two.

The exercises contained in this chapter are the following:

- Overhead Triceps Extension

- Skull Crusher

- Lying Triceps Extension

- Kick-Back

- Close Grip Press

- Standing Close Grip Press

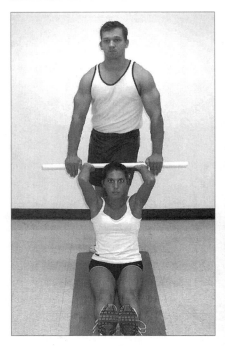
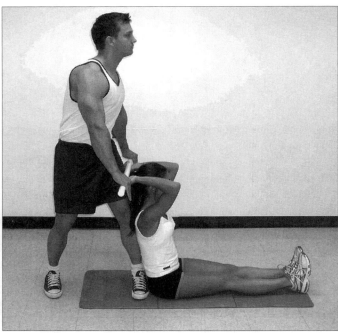

Fig. 9.1. Overhead triceps extension. Above: starting position. Below: finishing position.

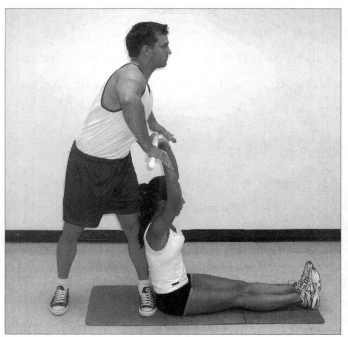
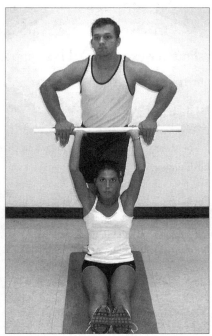

Overhead Triceps Extension

Introduction

- Primary muscle: triceps (back of the upper arm)

- Secondary muscle: forearms

- Movement: single-joint

- Performed: simultaneously with both arms

Trainer/Participant Position

(See Setup, pages 34–35.) The participant begins by sitting on the floor, keeping a straight back and upright posture. The trainer takes position behind the participant in a perpendicular fashion so that the side of the trainer's foot and leg are flat against the center of the participant's back. With the alternate leg, the trainer steps back slightly, creating a solid base for balance and for support of the participant's back. The participant should maintain a posture of a straight back with the chest out for the duration of the exercise.

In this position, the participant extends the arms upward so that they are perpendicular to the floor. Next, the participant rotates the upper arms back at the elbows until they are parallel to the ground. Using an overhand grip, the participant places his or her hands on the bar shoulder-width apart. Twisting at the waist, the trainer leans over the participant and positions his or her hands directly outside of the participant's hands with an open palm grip. The trainer's chest should be directly above the bar for leverage.

The Movement

The participant begins by pressing the bar upward in an arcing motion, rotating at the elbows. The arms are fully extended without locking the elbows. During the eccentric phase the participant slowly returns to the starting position, resisting the trainer. The movement is completed when the participant can no longer press upward. During the exercise, the arms must remain in the same position, shoulder-width apart. The only portion of the arms that move are the upper arms, which rotate at the elbows.

The trainer provides resistance by allowing the participant to push them up out of a slight leaning position to a standing one. During the eccentric phase, the trainer leans forward over the bar, pushing downward with the arms. The trainer creates leverage by keeping his or her body weight above the rotation point, which is in a fixed position. Additionally, the trainer is providing resistance at the point on the lever arm furthest from the point of rotation.

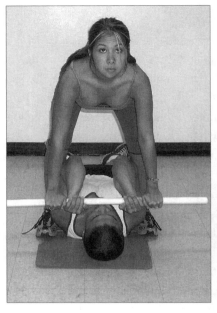
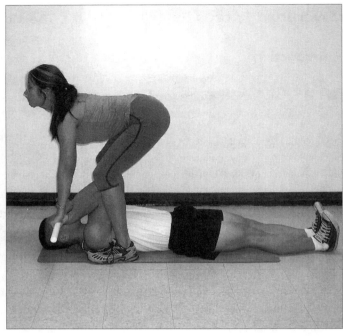

Fig. 9.2. Skull crushers. Above: starting position. Below: finishing position.

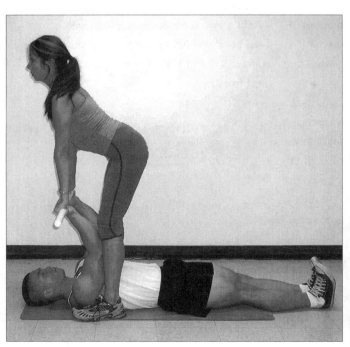
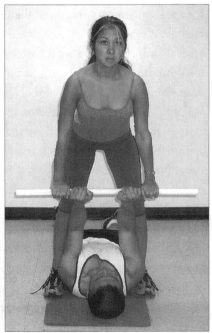

Skull Crushers

Introduction

- Primary muscle: triceps (back of the upper arm)

- Secondary muscle: forearm

- Movement: single-joint

- Performed: simultaneously with both arms

Trainer/Participant Position

The participant begins by lying down flat on his or her back on the floor. The arms, placed at the sides, are raised vertically toward the ceiling. Rotating back at the elbows, the arms form a 135-degree angle, with the hands just above the face. In this position, the arms (from the elbow to the shoulder) should be perpendicular to the body. The bar is gripped shoulder-width apart, with the palms facing away from the participant.

The trainer takes position by standing directly over the participant's upper chest. The trainer's feet are placed directly outside the participant's shoulders. This allows the participant's arms (from the shoulder to the elbow) to be locked in a fixed position, against the inner part of the trainer's lower legs. The trainer then squats down and leans over the participant in order to create leverage for resistance. Then, the trainer places his or her palms on the bar just outside of the participant's hands. It is important that the trainer keep his or her grip slightly loose and open in order to allow the bar to rotate freely on the palm during the movement.

The Movement

The participant begins the movement by extending the upper arms upward in an arcing motion, rotating at the elbows. The arms are fully extended, without locking the elbows. During the eccentric phase, the participant slowly returns to the starting position, resisting the trainer. Repeat this until the triceps muscles reach exhaustion. Arm rotation should only occur at the elbow joint, not the shoulder.

The trainer provides the resistance by allowing the participant to push them up, slightly out of the squatting position during the concentric phase. During the eccentric phase, the trainer squats back down, pressing down with the arms. The trainer maintains a leverage advantage as his or her body weight is above the axis of rotation (the participant's elbows). It is important that the trainer keeps his or her arms extended, allowing most of the resistance to be provided by his or her own body weight.

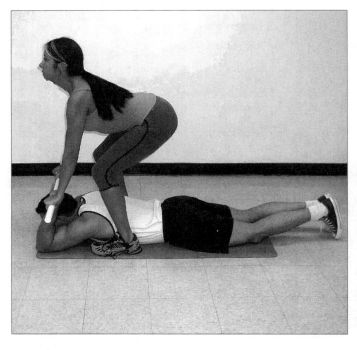

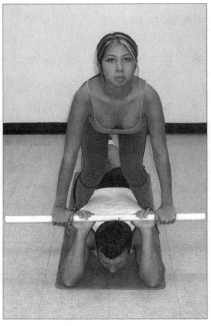

Fig. 9.3. Lying triceps extension.
Above: starting position.
Below: finishing position.

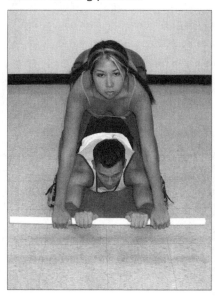

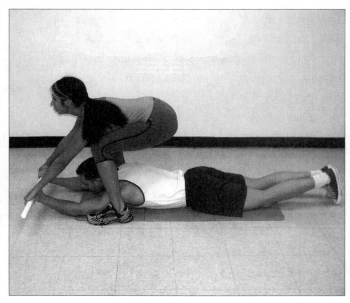

Lying Triceps Extension

Introduction

- Primary muscle: triceps (back of the upper arm)

- Secondary muscle: forearms

- Movement: single-joint

- Performed: simultaneously with both arms

Trainer/Participant Position

The participant begins by lying face down on the floor. The participant then extends the arms in front of the body, shoulder-width apart. Finally, the arms are rotated upward at the elbow to a 90-degree angle (perpendicular to the floor). The bar is gripped shoulder-width apart, with the palms facing away from the participant.

The trainer takes position by squatting down over the participant's upper back, so that the feet are placed just outside of the participant's shoulders. With an open palm, the trainer then positions his or her hands on the bar just outside of the participant's hands. The grip should remain loose enough to allow the bar to roll along the hands during the movement.

The Movement

The participant begins the movement by pressing the bar toward the ground, rotating at the elbows. The arms should fully extend, without locking. During the eccentric phase of the movement, the participant slowly returns to the starting position, resisting the trainer. The movement is repeated until the triceps are completely fatigued.

The trainer, beginning in a squatting position, provides resistance by allowing the participant to pull the trainer's body into more of an upright position. During the eccentric motion, the trainer returns to a squatting position, pulling the bar back to the starting point. A leverage advantage is gained as the trainer is positioned higher than the triceps, allowing gravity to do much of the work.

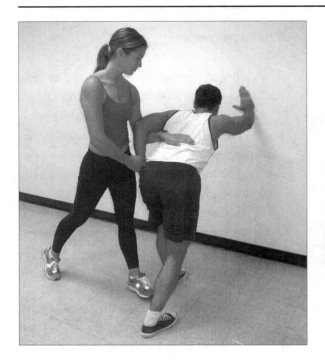

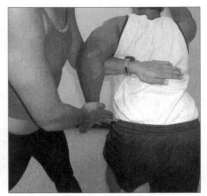

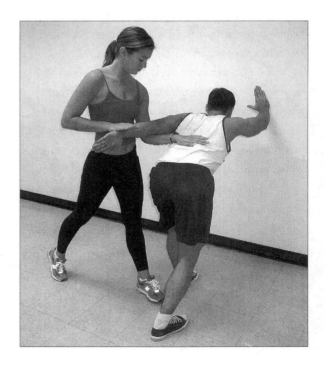

Fig. 9.4. Kick-back.
Above right: hand position
Above left: starting position.
Bottom right: finishing position.

Kick-Back

Introduction

- Primary muscle: triceps (back of the upper arm)

- Secondary muscle: not applicable

- Movement: single-joint

- Performed: one arm at a time

Trainer/Participant Position

The participant begins by facing a wall, standing one to two feet away. The participant then leans forward at the waist until the chest is parallel to the floor. The feet should be positioned shoulder-width apart and offset for balance. One hand is placed with the palm flat against the wall for stability. The other arm is positioned along the side of the body, bent 90 degrees at the elbow. The upper arm is raised up until the elbow is about 6 inches above the back.

The trainer takes position by standing next to the participant's side with his or her feet off set facing the participant's side. Then, the trainer places the arm closest to the wall under the participant's raised arm at the elbow. The trainer's forearm and hand rest flat along the participant's mid-back. The trainer takes his or her opposite hand and places it firmly, with an open palm, just above the participant's wrist.

The Movement

The participant begins the movement by extending the lower arm, rotating at the elbow. The arm is parallel to the ground, fully extended, without locking the elbow. During the eccentric phase, the participant slowly returns to the starting position, resisting the trainer. Repeat this movement, until the triceps are completely exhausted.

The trainer provides resistance by pressing the palm of the hand against the extension of the participant's arm. During the eccentric phase, the trainer presses the participant's arm down in an arcing motion back to the starting point. The trainer maintains leverage by placing the palm of the hand at the furthest point on the lever arm (above the wrist), away from the point of rotation. In order to gain more leverage, the trainer can position themselves facing toward the same direction as the participant. Additionally, the trainer can increase leverage by moving his or her body closer to the participant's body.

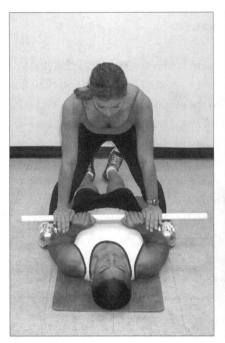
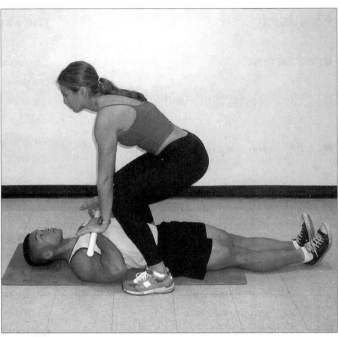

Fig. 9.3. Close grip press. Above: starting position. Below: finishing position.

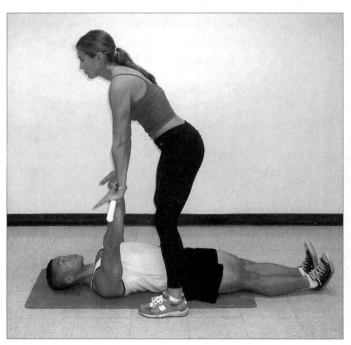
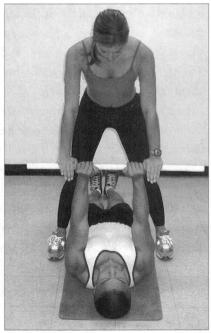

Close Grip Press

Introduction

- Primary muscle: triceps (back of the upper arms)

- Secondary muscle: pectoralis (chest)

- Movement: multi-joint

- Performed: simultaneous arm movement

Trainer/Participant Position

The participant begins by lying down flat on his or her back with the legs and feet together. The arms are placed directly at the sides, with the triceps (back of the arm) resting on the floor. The elbows are then rotated upward to a 90-degree angle so that the upper arm is perpendicular to the floor. The participant then takes an overhand grip on the bar, shoulder-width apart.

The trainer takes position by standing directly over the participant's abdomen with the feet just outside and below the participant's arms. Then the trainer squats down and places his or her hands just outside of the participant's grip. The trainer's arms should be straight and in a vertical plane perpendicular to the floor. The trainer's chest is positioned directly above the bar in order to gain leverage and provide smooth resistance during the exercise.

The Movement

The exercise begins as the participant presses straight upward in a vertical motion. The arms are extended until nearly straight without locking the elbows. During the eccentric phase the participant returns slowly to the starting position, resisting the trainer. The movement is completed when the triceps reach complete exhaustion. In order to isolate the triceps, the arms should remain shoulder-width apart and close to the side of the body throughout the duration of the exercise.

The trainer provides resistance by allowing his or her body to be pushed from a squatting stance to more of an upright position during the concentric phase of the movement. During the eccentric phase the trainer returns to the squatting position, pressing downward. The trainer gains leverage by keeping his or her chest directly above the bar and the arms in an extended position. Resistance is provided by the trainer's own body weight and gravity.

111

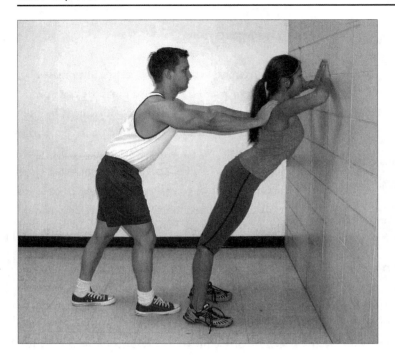

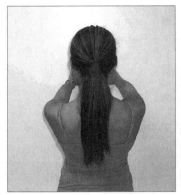

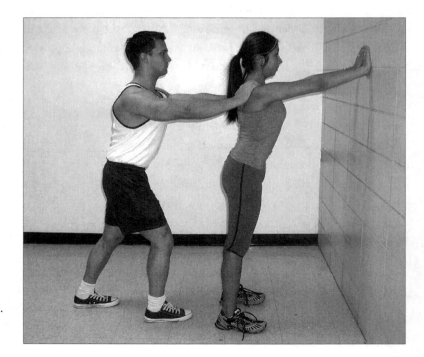

Fig. 9.6. Close grip wall press.
Above right: setup position
Above left: starting position.
Bottom right: finishing position.

Close Grip Wall Press

Introduction

- Primary muscle: triceps (back of the upper arm)

- Secondary muscles: pectoralis major (chest), and posterior deltoid (back of the shoulder)

- Movement: multi-joint

- Performed: simultaneously with both arms

Trainer/Participant Position

The participant begins by facing a wall and stands a little more than an arm's length away with his or her feet shoulder-width apart. The arms are extended and raised until the hands reach eye level. The palms are placed flat against the wall, side by side. Keeping the feet flat on the floor, the participant leans forward until the face is directly in front of the hands.

The trainer takes position by standing an arm's length away from the participant. The feet are shoulder-width apart and in an offset stance. Then, the trainer extends his or her arms and leans forward to place the palms of the hands flat on the participant's shoulder blades.

The Movement

The participant begins by pressing outward from the wall. The arms are fully extended without locking the elbows. During the eccentric phase, the participant slowly returns to the starting position, resisting the trainer. The movement is repeated until the triceps reach complete exhaustion. The trainer provides resistance by leaning forward, allowing the participant to push the trainer's body back. During the eccentric phase, the trainer leans forward, taking a step if necessary and pushing with the arms. The trainer maintains leverage by leaning his or her body forward, causing the participant to absorb the weight. As the participant's arms are extended, the participant significantly reduces the trainer's mechanical advantage. But as the participant gets closer to the wall, they will lose that mechanical advantage and the movement will become increasingly difficult.

10.

Exercises for the Biceps

This chapter deals with the second muscle group for the upper arm, the biceps. The bicep group is the primary elbow flexor and is also used in shoulder flexion. Although the muscles of the tricep group are much stronger, those of the bicep group contract with more speed than the triceps.

Here is a list of the exercises contained in this chapter:

■ Biceps Curl

■ Lying Biceps Curl

■ Preacher Curl

■ One-Arm Isolation Curl

■ Reverse Curl

■ Concentration Curl

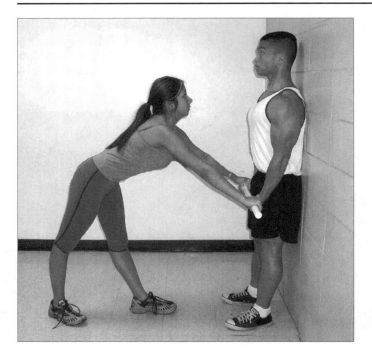

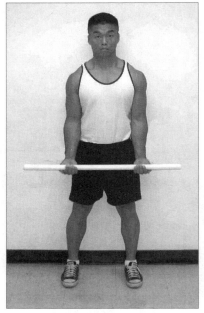

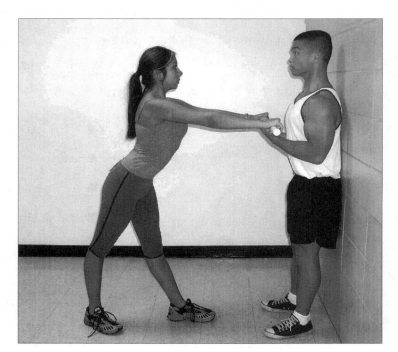

Fig. 10.1. Biceps curl.
Above right: setup position
Above left: starting position.
Bottom right: finishing
position.

Biceps Curl

Introduction

- Primary muscle: biceps (front of the upper arm)

- Secondary muscle: forearms

- Movement: single-joint

- Performed: simultaneous motion with both arms

Trainer/Participant Position

The participant begins by standing with his or her back flat against a wall or stable surface. The feet are positioned shoulder-width apart and slightly away from the wall to provide stability. The arms are extended down by the participant's rib cage with the back of the arms firmly placed against the sides of the body. Using an underhand grip, the participant firmly grasps the bar.

The trainer takes position by facing the participant. The trainer should stand one to two feet away in an offset stance with the feet shoulder-width apart. Bending at the waist, the trainer leans forward, and grasps the bar directly outside the participant's hands with an open palm. The grip should remain loose enough to allow the hands to roll along the bar through the movement of the exercise.

The Movement

The participant begins by curling the bar upward toward the chest in an arcing motion, rotating at the elbows. The movement should continue to 135 degrees, until the bar is a few inches from the chest. During the eccentric phase the bar is slowly lowered back to the starting position, resisting the trainer. Repeat this movement until the biceps reach exhaustion. The wrists should remain in a straight line with the forearm throughout the movement, ensuring the resistance is concentrated on the biceps.

The trainer provides resistance by allowing the participant to push the trainer's body upward from a leaning position to more of a standing one. During the eccentric phase the trainer presses down, returning to a leaning position. A leverage advantage is maintained as the trainer's chest and shoulder (the center of gravity) remain above the participant's elbow.

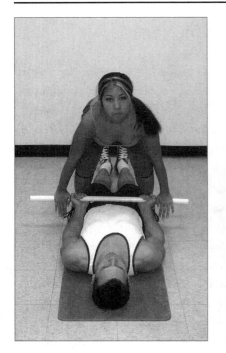
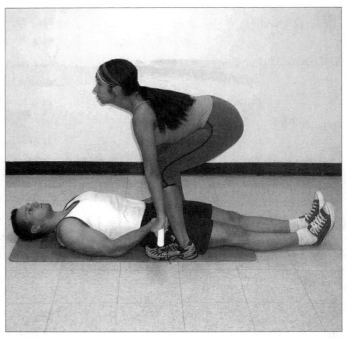

Fig. 10.2. Lying biceps curl. Above: starting position. Below: finishing position.

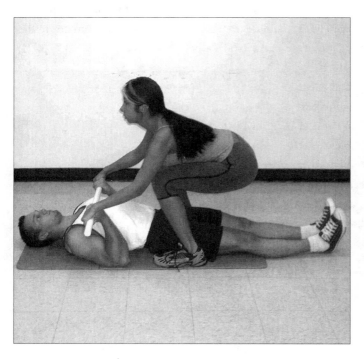
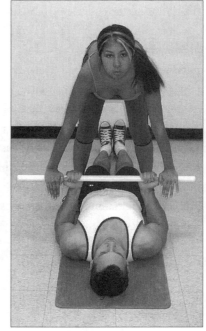

Lying Biceps Curl

Introduction

- Primary muscle: biceps (front of the upper arm)

- Secondary muscle: forearms

- Movement: single-joint

- Performed: simultaneously with both arms

Trainer/Participant Position

The participant begins by lying down flat on his or her back on the floor. The legs and feet are positioned together, flat on the floor. The arms are placed at the sides of the body with the palm facing up. The participant then takes a firm grip on the bar with the hands shoulder-width apart.

The trainer takes position by squatting down over the participant's upper thighs and waist. The trainer's feet are placed just below the participant's hands on either side of the body. The trainer then reaches forward and grasps the bar overhand with the palms of the hands directly outside the hands of the participant. The bar should remain slightly loose in the palm of the trainer's hand to allow for rotation during the movement.

The Movement

The participant begins by curling the bar upward toward the chest in an arcing motion, rotating at the elbows. The bar should continue to 135 degrees until it is a few inches from the chest. During the eccentric phase the bar is slowly returned to the starting position, resisting the trainer. Repeat this movement until the biceps are exhausted. The wrists should remain in a straight line with the forearms throughout the movement, ensuring the resistance is concentrated on the biceps.

The trainer provides resistance by allowing the participant to pull the trainer's body slightly up during the movement and back down again as the bar reaches the 135-degree angle. During the eccentric phase, the trainer pulls the bar back to the starting position, moving his or her body upward with the arc or the movement and back down at completion. It is necessary for the trainer to use some arm strength during the exercise. Leverage is attained by standing over the participant and moving along the line of the arc during the movement.

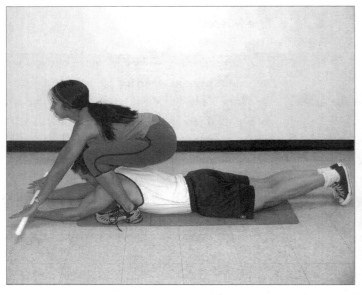

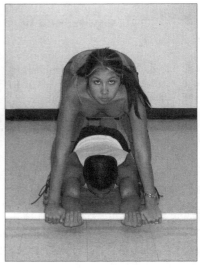

Fig. 10.3. Preacher curl.
Above: starting position.
Below: finishing position.

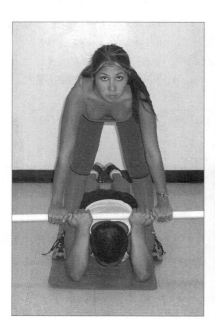

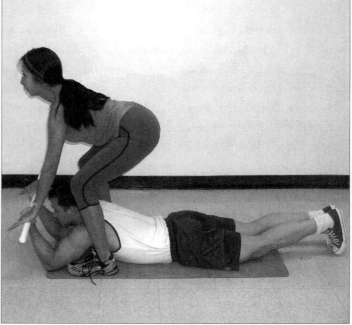

Preacher Curl

Introduction

- Primary muscle: biceps (front of the upper arms)

- Secondary muscle: forearms

- Movement: single-joint

- Performed: simultaneously with both arms

Trainer/Participant Position

The participant begins by lying face down on the floor. The participant then extends the arms in front of the body, shoulder-width apart. The hands are placed shoulder-width apart on the bar, using an underhand grip.

The trainer takes position by squatting down over the participant's upper back, so that the feet are placed just outside of the participant's shoulders. With an open palm, the trainer then positions his or her hands on the bar just outside of the participant's hands. The grip should remain loose enough to allow the bar to roll along the hands during the movement.

The Movement

The participant begins the movement by curling the bar upward toward the head in an arcing motion, rotating at the elbows. The movement should continue until the bar is a few inches from the head, just past 90 degrees. During the eccentric phase, the participant slowly returns to the starting position, resisting the trainer. The movement is repeated until the biceps are completely fatigued.

The trainer, beginning in a squatting position, provides resistance by allowing the participant to pull the trainer's body into more of an upright position. During the eccentric motion, the trainer returns to a squatting position, pushing the bar back down to the starting point. A leverage advantage is gained as the trainer is positioned higher than the rotation point of the biceps, allowing gravity to do much of the work.

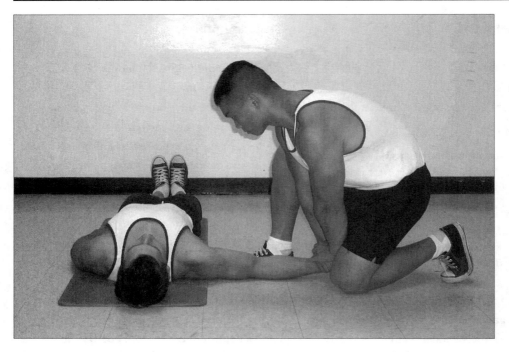

Fig. 10.4. One-arm isolation curl. Above: starting position. Below: finishing position.

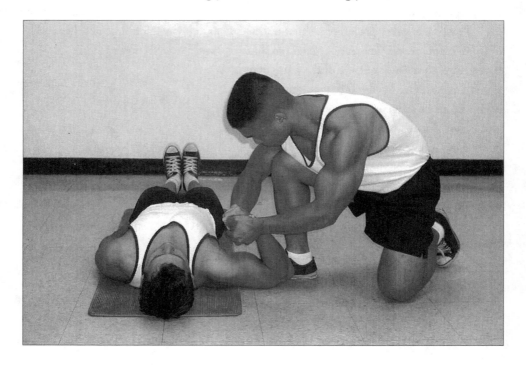

One-Arm Isolation Curl

Introduction

- Primary muscle: biceps (front of the upper arm)

- Secondary muscle: forearm

- Movement: single-joint

- Performed: one arm at a time

Trainer/Participant Position

The participant begins by lying down flat on his or her back. The legs and feet are positioned together and remain straight. The arms are rotated upward so that they are on the same plane as the shoulders. The non-working hand on the opposite side is placed palm down on the floor for balance and stability. The working hand on the trainer side is faced palm up.

The trainer takes position by kneeling down, facing the participant's side at the elbow. The trainer places the forward foot along the participant's elbow and upper arm for stability. The trainer reaches down and grips the participant's hand at the thumb and then places his or her other hand directly on top of both.

The Movement

The participant begins by curling the biceps upward, rotating at the elbow, up to 135 degrees. During the eccentric phase, the participant slowly returns to the starting position (0 degrees) resisting the trainer. This movement is repeated until the biceps reach exhaustion. The wrist should remain straight and in line with the forearm so that the resistance remains constant on the biceps.

The trainer provides resistance by pulling against the upward arc of the movement. During the eccentric phase, the trainer pulls the participant's arm down through the arc of the movement to the starting position. The trainer maintains a leverage advantage by placing resistance at the furthest point of the lever arm away from the rotation (the wrist). Additionally, the participant's arm is isolated by the floor and the trainer's foot, allowing the trainer to place his or her center of gravity over the lever arm.

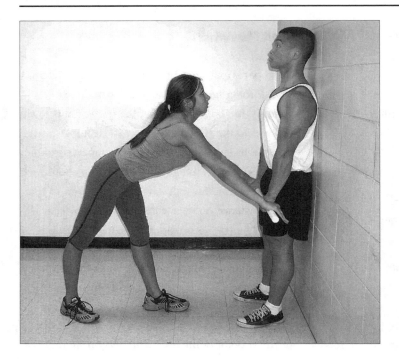

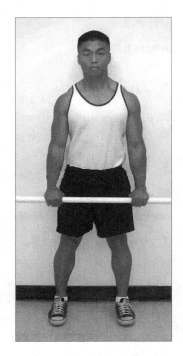

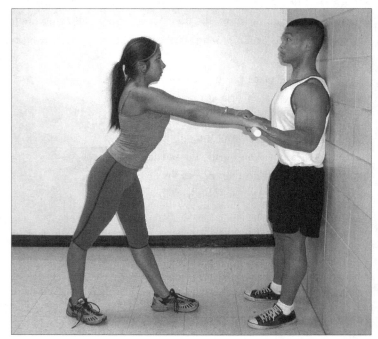

Fig. 10.5. Reverse curl.
Above right: setup position
Above left: starting position.
Bottom right: finishing
position.

Reverse Curl

Introduction

- Primary muscle: forearms

- Secondary muscle: biceps (front of the upper arm)

- Movement: single-joint

- Performed: simultaneously with both arms

Trainer/Participant Position

The participant begins by standing with his or her back flat against a wall or stable surface. The feet are positioned shoulder-width apart and slightly away from the wall to provide stability. The arms are extended down by the participant's rib cage with the back of the arms firmly placed against the sides of the body. Using an overhand grip, the participant firmly grasps the bar.

The trainer takes position by facing the participant. The trainer should stand one to two feet away in an offset stance with the feet shoulder-width apart. Bending at the waist, the trainer leans forward, and grasps the bar directly outside the participant's hands with an open palm. The grip should remain loose enough to allow the hands to roll along the bar through the movement of the exercise.

The Movement

The participant begins by curling the bar upward toward the chest in an arcing motion, rotating at the elbows. The movement should continue to 135 degrees, until the bar is a few inches from the chest. During the eccentric phase the bar is slowly lowered back to the starting position, resisting the trainer. Repeat this movement until the biceps reach exhaustion. Throughout the movement, the wrists should remain in a straight line with the forearm, ensuring the resistance is concentrated on the biceps.

The trainer provides resistance by allowing the participant to push the trainer's body upward from a leaning position to more of a standing one. During the eccentric phase the trainer presses down, returning to a leaning position. A leverage advantage is maintained as the trainer's chest and shoulder (the center of gravity) remain above the participant's elbow.

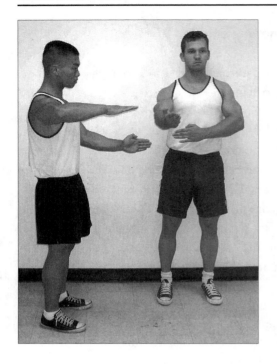

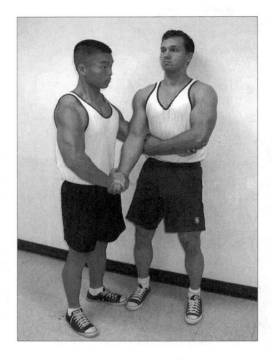

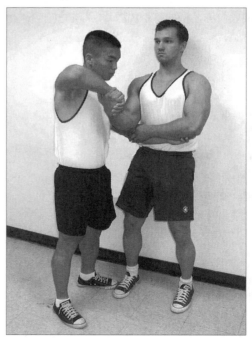

Fig. 10.6. Concentration curl.
Above left: setup position
Above right: starting position.
Bottom right: finishing
position.

Concentration Curl

Introduction

- Primary muscle: biceps (front of the upper arm)

- Secondary muscle: forearms

- Movement: single-joint

- Performed: one arm at a time (trainer-participant using the right arm for this demonstration)

Participant Position (before Trainer/Participant interlock)

The participant elevates his or her extended left arm up to the ceiling and places the 90-degree bent arm across the stomach with the under side of the forearm facing the stomach. The participant must leave a little space between the forearm and the stomach for the trainer to place his or her forearm.

Trainer Position (before Trainer/Participant interlock)

The trainer faces the participant's right arm and raises his or her extended left arm parallel to the shoulders. Then, the trainer bends his or her right arm, bent 90 degrees, along the side of the rib cage with the hands open, parallel to the participant's body.

Trainer/Participant Position (interlock)

The participant lowers his or her right-extended arm until it reaches the back of the participant's left hand. The left hand grasps the trainer's left forearm. The right palm is on the trainer's right palm while the hands interlock.

The trainer steps forward, and slides his or her left forearm between the participant's left forearm and stomach. The left hand grasps the participant's left forearm. The left arm is lowered to the rib cage and the palms are placed against participant's palms. The hands are interlocked.

The Movement

The participant begins by curling the arm upward to the chest, rotating at the elbow. During the eccentric phase, the participant slowly returns to the starting position, resisting the trainer. The movement is repeated until the biceps reach exhaustion.

The trainer provides resistance by pressing against the participant's hand in the opposite direction of the rotation. During the eccentric phase, the trainer presses downward against the participant's hand in an arcing motion, down to the starting point. The resistance is provided by the trainer's chest, triceps, and oblique. Leverage is gained as the trainer keeps the participant's arm isolated in a fixed position, with the resistance at the end of the lever arm. Greater leverage can be obtained by turning to face the participant, allowing greater use of the chest and shoulder.

11.

Exercises for the Glutes

Unlike many other muscle groups, the glutes are almost entirely made up of one large muscle — the gluteus maximus, and are supported by several other smaller muscles. The activity most associated with the glutes is the extension of the legs as they move backward and also as they move laterally (i.e., toward the side). The hip joint, associated closely with the glutes, is a true ball and socket joint and therefore does not have the same range of motion associated with the shoulder but is far more stable. All lower body power originates from the glutes and this makes it highly applicable to most sports.

Only two exercises apply to this muscle group, as follows:

- Glute Raises

- Butt Kick

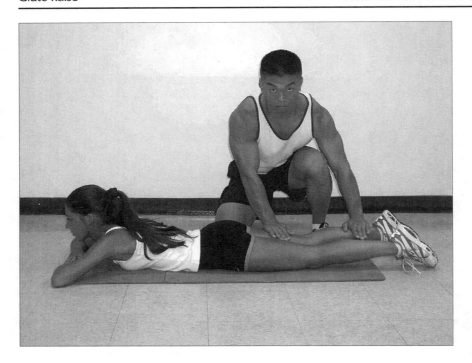

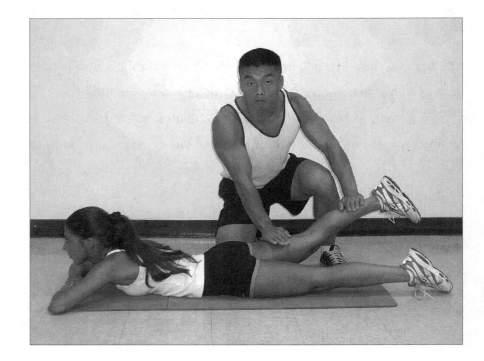

Fig. 11.1. Glute
raise.
Above: starting
position.
Right: finishing
position.

Glute Raise

Introduction

- Primary muscle: glutes (buttocks)

- Secondary muscle: hamstrings (back of the upper leg)

- Movement: single-joint

- Performed: one leg at a time

Trainer/Participant Position

The participant begins the exercise by lying face down on the floor. The hands are placed under the chin or in the most comfortable position for the participant. The participant's legs are set slightly apart and remain that way for the duration of the exercise.

The trainer begins by kneeling at one side of the participant, next to the legs. The trainer selects a leg and places one hand at the mid-thigh and the other directly on the calf. The trainer's hands should be placed firmly at these points with the palms flat against the leg.

The Movement

Keeping the leg straight, the participant rotates the leg upward at the hip, squeezing the glute. The participant should rotate the leg upward as high as possible in order to achieve a full range of motion. The participant then resists the movement back to the starting position and repeats as the leg touches the floor. It is important for the participant to keep the leg straight throughout the duration of the exercise. Any bend in the knee will cause a break in the movement, and a loss of isolation.

The trainer, kneeling beside the participant, provides resistance by pushing against the upward movement of the leg. During the eccentric motion the trainer pushes the participant's leg downward toward the floor. The small range of motion and the trainer's position above the participant's leg provide a dramatic leverage advantage for the trainer.

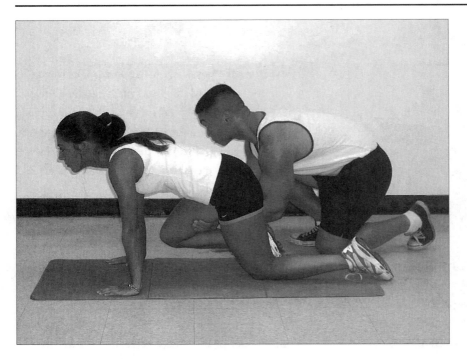

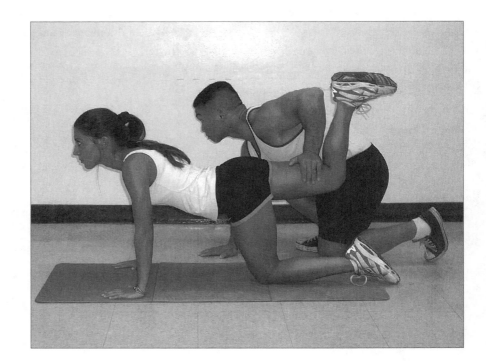

Fig. 11.2. Butt kick.
Above: starting position.
Right: finishing position.

Butt Kick

Introduction

■   This exercise primarily benefits the gluteus
(buttocks) with secondary work being
performed by the hamstrings (back of the
legs).

Trainer/Participant Position

The participant begins the exercise by kneeling
down on the ground, with the knees shoulder-
width apart. The participant places the palms of
his or her hands flat on the ground, shoulder-
width apart. The participant's arms remain
straight and should be perpendicular to the
ground in this position. The back remains straight
and the chest out throughout the exercise.

   The trainer assumes a kneeling position on
one side of the participant, so that they are both
facing the same direction. The trainer should be
positioned as close to the side of the participant as
possible in order to maximize leverage. With one
hand firmly on the ground for support, the trainer
then firmly places an open palm on the back of
the participant's leg near the back of the knee.

The Movement

Beginning the exercise in the starting position, the
participant brings the leg forward, so that the
knee is under the chest. The back will bend
slightly in this position. After the knee is brought
under the chest, the participant kicks back and
upward, squeezing the glute. The leg continues
back and upward until the thigh becomes parallel
to the ground. During the eccentric phase, the
participant slowly returns to the starting position,
resisting the trainer. The movement is completed
when the participant reaches fatigue.

   The trainer provides resistance by pushing
the participant's knee under the chest at the start
and then allowing the participant to kick back and
upward. During the eccentric movement, the
trainer pushes the participant's leg down and forward, returning the knee under the chest. The
trainer is able to provide resistance by positioning
his or her body close to the body of the participant and facing the same direction. As long as
the trainer's shoulder and upper arm remain
above the participant's leg, a leverage advantage
is present.

12.

Exercises for the Abdominals

The abdominals are comprised of the rectus abdominus, the internal obliques, and the external obliques. The abdominals have an extremely high level of muscular endurance but conversely have a very low level of muscular strength. The abdominals run from the lower portion of the chest down to the pelvis. The primary function of the abdominals is to bring the pelvis closer to the rib cage and vice versa.

The exercises contained in this chapter are the following:

- Boxer Crunch

- Oblique Crunch

- Power Crunch

- Resisted Crunch

- Reverse Crunch

- Pelvic Thrust

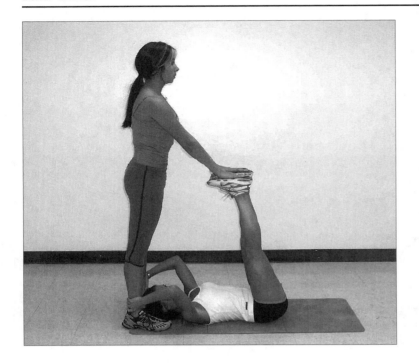

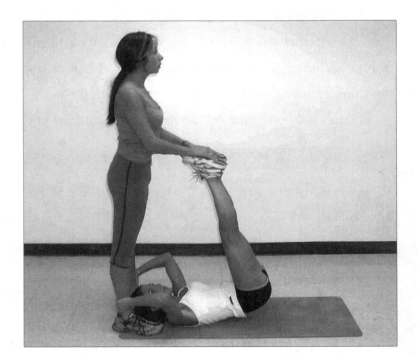

Fig. 12.1. Boxer crunch.
Above: starting position.
Right: finishing position.

Boxer Crunch

Introduction

- Primary muscle: obliques (sides of the abdomen)

- Secondary muscle: overall abdomen

- Movement: single-joint

- Performed: one motion

Trainer/Participant Position

The participant begins by lying on his or her back and then reaches back to grasp the trainer's ankles once the trainer moves into position. With the head between the trainer's feet, the participant raises his or her legs perpendicular to the floor with the knees slightly bent. The feet remain as flat as possible and parallel to the floor in order to give the trainer an even surface in order to place his or her hands.

The trainer stands with his or her feet just out side of the participant's ears. The trainer then places his or her palms on the heels of the participant to provide the greatest amount of stability. The fingers are place around the heel to prevent slipping. The forearms are placed along the bottom of the participant's feet to provide stability.

The Movement

The participant begins by raising the lower body off of the floor, pushing the legs vertically toward the ceiling and in a slight arc toward the trainer. This will cause the pelvis and the lower back to elevate off the ground, bringing the pelvis up toward the rib cage. During the eccentric phase the lower back and pelvis are returned to the original resting position. The movement is completed when the participant can no longer raise the lower body off of the floor.

The trainer provides resistance by pressing down on the soles of the participant's shoes as the participant's legs raise upward. During the eccentric phase the trainer presses downward toward the floor. The trainer has a natural leverage advantage because the participant's feet are below the height of the trainer's shoulders. It is important that the trainer provides a steady amount of resistance through out the movement to prevent a break in the movement and possible injury to the lower back.

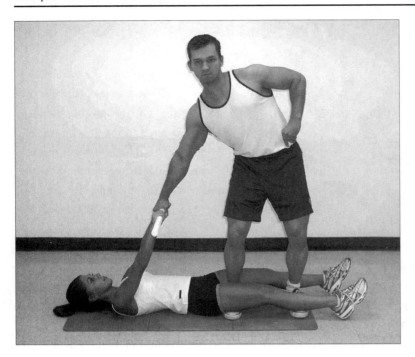

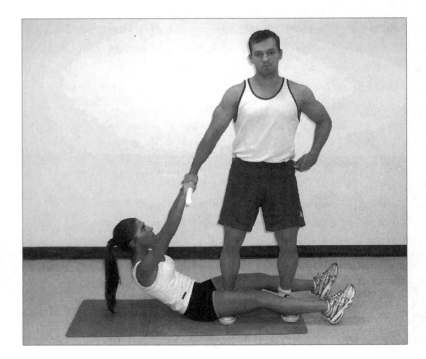

Fig. 12.2. Oblique crunch.
Above: starting position.
Right: finishing position.

Oblique Crunch

Introduction

- Primary muscle: obliques (sides of the abdominals)

- Secondary muscles: abdominals

- Movement: single-joint

- Performed: one side at a time

Trainer/Participant Position

The participant begins by assuming a standing position, with the feet shoulder-width apart for stability. The participant grips the bar at its center with one hand. The arms remain at the participant's sides so that the bar is parallel to the floor.

After the participant is in position, the trainer approaches the same side of the body as the bar. The trainer then sits down, with one leg over the participant's feet and the other behind the heels. Reaching up the trainer firmly grasps the bar directly outside the participant's hand. Next, the trainer leans backward, pulling the participant over, so that they are leaning at the hips.

The Movement

Beginning from the leaning position, the participant straightens up to the standing position. During the eccentric phase, the participant slowly and carefully returns to the leaning position, lowering the trainer's body weight. The movement is completed when the participant is unable to straighten into a standing position.

The trainer provides resistance with his or her own body weight. During the concentric movement, the trainer allows the participant to pull them up toward a sitting position. During the eccentric phase, the trainer slowly leans back toward the ground, pulling the participant with them. The trainer creates leverage by pulling from the furthest point on the lever arm, away from the point of rotation.

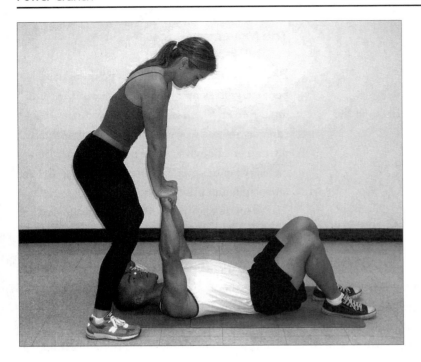

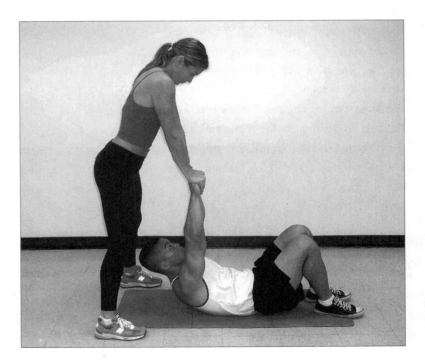

Fig. 12.3. Power crunch.
Above: starting position.
Right: finishing position.

Power Crunch

Introduction

- Primary muscle: abdominals

- Secondary muscle: not applicable

- Movement: single-joint

- Performed: one motion

Trainer/Participant Position

The participant begins by lying down flat on his or her back. With the knees bent in a 45-degree angle, the feet are firmly placed on the ground to provide stability and prevent the body from slipping back and forth. Making a fist with each hand, the participant extends the arms upward, perpendicular to the floor and positions the hands side by side.

The trainer takes position by standing with the feet shoulder-width apart, outside of the participant's ears. The trainer, bending slightly at the knees, leans over slightly and grasps the participant's fists. In this position, the trainer's chest and hands should be directly over the participant's arms, creating a leverage advantage.

The Movement

The participant begins the movement from the starting position by "crunching" forward towards the thighs until the shoulders come off of the ground. The arms, which remain straight, rotate forward in a slight arc through the motion. During the eccentric phase, the participant slowly lowers the upper body to its original position, against the resistance of the trainer. Repeat this movement until the desired level of exercise is reached.

The trainer provides resistance by pushing straight down through the participant's arms. The same holds true during the eccentric phase of the exercise. Leverage is provided as the trainer's center of gravity (the chest) is placed over the participant's arms. If the trainer needs to gain leverage, the feet can be positioned closer to the participant's shoulders. This will allow the trainer to transfer more of his or her body weight onto the participant.

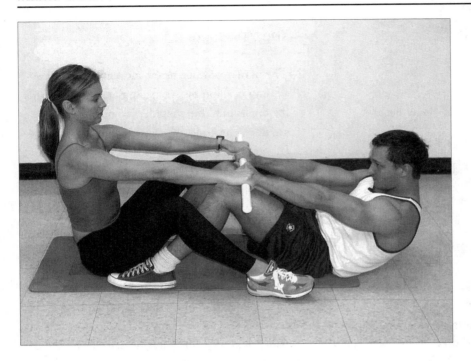

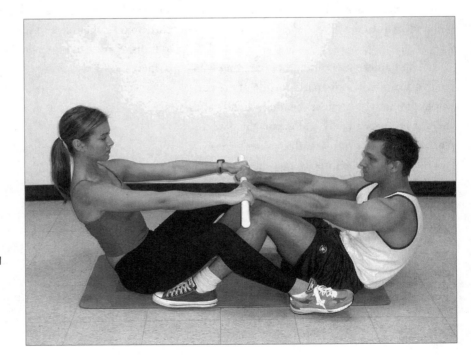

Fig. 12.4. Resisted
crunch.
Above: starting
position.
Right: finishing
position.

Resisted Crunch

Introduction

- Primary muscle: abdominals

- Secondary muscle: not applicable

- Movement: single-joint

- Performed: one motion

Trainer/Participant Position

The participant begins by sitting on the floor with the knees bent at a 45-degree angle. The feet are placed firmly on the floor shoulder-width apart forming a solid base. The participant then assumes a "crunched" position.

The trainer assumes a seated position directly facing the participant. The trainer then moves forward and interlocks legs with the participant for support, with the trainer's legs on the outside. The trainer's feet are placed on the floor directly outside the participant's hips and the trainer's knees are directly outside the participant's knees. The trainer takes an overhand grip on the bar shoulder-width apart and places it just past the participant's knees. The participant places his or her hands just inside the trainers, keeping the arms straight.

The Movement

The participant begins in the crunched position by pressing the bar forward, just past the knees. During the eccentric phase, the participant resists as the trainer pushes the bar slowly back over the knees to the starting point. Repeat this movement until the desired exercise level is achieved. The participant's arms remain straight throughout the duration of the exercise.

The trainer provides resistance by pressing against the bar as the pushes it over the knees. During the eccentric phase, the trainer pushes the bar back over the knees to the starting point. The trainer maintains leverage as the point of resistance remains above the abdominals.

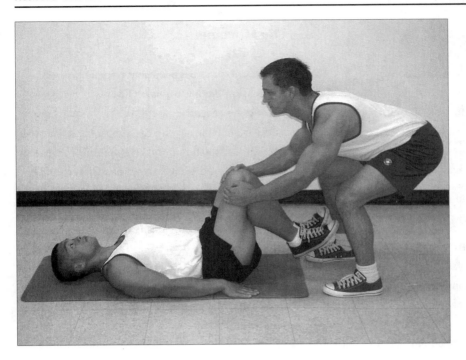

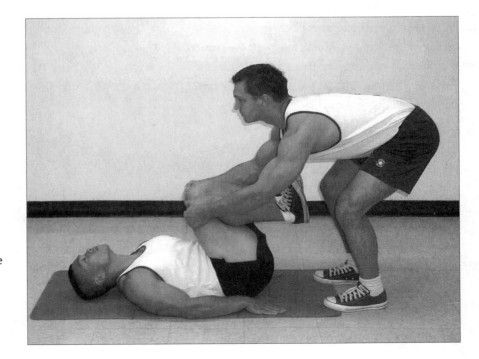

Fig. 12.5. Reverse crunch.
Above: starting position.
Right: finishing position.

Resisted Crunch

Introduction

- Primary muscle: abdominals

- Secondary muscle: hip flexors (hip girdle)

- Movement: single-joint

- Performed: one motion

Trainer/Participant Position

The participant begins by lying down flat on his or her back on the floor. The legs are raised and bent at the knees to form a 90-degree angle. In this position, the upper leg (from the knee to the hip) is perpendicular to the floor. The arms are placed at the sides with the hands on the floor, palms down, for stability.

The trainer takes position by standing directly in front of the participant's feet. Squatting down, the trainer places his or her hands on the participant's legs, just above the knees.

Movement

The participant begins by pulling the knees from the starting position (with the upper leg perpendicular to the floor) as close to the chest as possible. During the eccentric phase, the participant slowly returns to the starting position, resisting the trainer. The movement is repeated until the desired exercise level is achieved. It is important that the participant not return the legs beyond the starting point. Moving down beyond the starting point would cause the lower back to work, possibly causing injury.

The trainer provides resistance by resisting with the arms as the participant pulls the knees toward the chest. During the eccentric phase, the trainer pulls the participant's legs back to the starting point (with the upper leg perpendicular to the floor). The trainer needs to carefully monitor the participant's form, making sure the legs do not move lower than the starting position. Little leverage or strength is required by the trainer in order to provide resistance. This is largely due to the limited strength of the abdominal muscle.

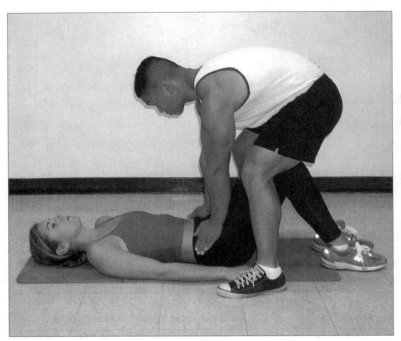

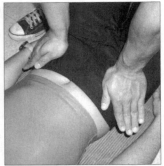

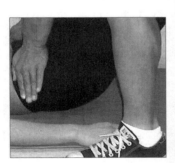

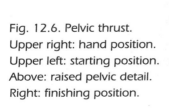

Fig. 12.6. Pelvic thrust.
Upper right: hand position.
Upper left: starting position.
Above: raised pelvic detail.
Right: finishing position.

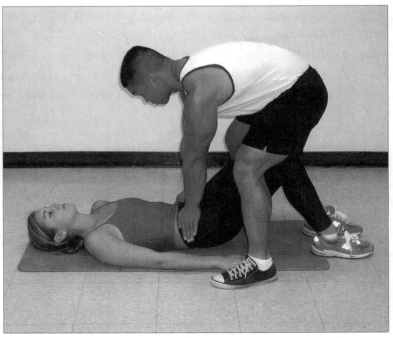

Pelvic Thrust

Introduction

- Primary muscle: hip flexors (hip girdle)

- Secondary muscle: abdominals

- Movement: single-joint

- Performed: one motion

Trainer/Participant Position

The participant begins by lying down flat on his or her back. The knees are bent at a 45-degree angle and the feet are placed flat on the ground. The arms are placed slightly outward from the sides with the palms flat against the ground to help provide stability.

The trainer stands directly over the participant's thighs with his or her feet just outside the participant's legs. Squatting down, the trainer places a hand on each hip. The arms should be extended, forming a vertical line to the participant's waist. The chest must be directly above the hips in order to gain leverage and provide a smooth resistance during the exercise.

The Movement

The exercise begins as the participant raises the hips upward and the buttocks off of the ground toward the ceiling. During the eccentric phase, the participant slowly lowers the hips and buttock back to the ground, resisting the trainer. Repeat this movement until the hip flexors reach complete exhaustion. The feet and back remain flat on the floor throughout the exercise

The trainer provides resistance by allowing the participant to push them slightly up out of the initial squatting stance during the concentric motion. During the eccentric phase, the trainer returns to the squatting position, pushing downward toward the floor. The trainer gains leverage by keeping his or her chest directly above the participant's waist and the arms in an extended position.

13.

Exercises for the Wrists

The wrist functions to enable four essential movements, which are performed by a combination of two primary muscle groups. These muscle groups are referred to as the wrist flexors and wrist extensors. There are also several muscles which control the digits (fingers) but are also used as secondary movers of the wrist joint. The wrist muscles are often used to stabilize the bar or the resistance throughout many other exercises in the book.

There aren't many exercises you can do with the wrist. Consequently, only a single exercise will be described in this chapter:

■ Wrist Curl

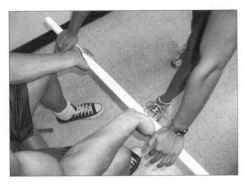

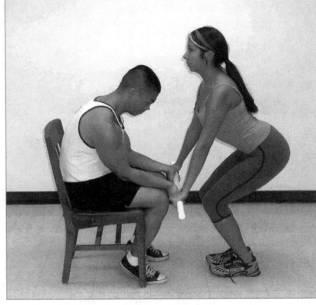

Figs. 13.1. Wrist curl.
Top left: hand position
Right: starting position
Below: finishing position.

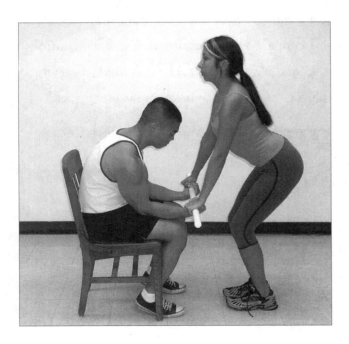

Wrist Curl

Introduction

■ Primary muscles: forearms, wrists

■ Secondary muscles: not applicable

■ Movement: single-joint

■ Performed: simultaneously with both arms

Trainer/Participant Position

The participant begins the exercise by sitting in a sturdy chair. The feet are placed firmly on the floor, shoulder-width apart. Leaning over, the participant rests his or her arms directly on top of the legs, with the wrists over the edge of the knees. The bar is gripped underhand, with the wrists bent in a down (extended) position.

The trainer takes position by standing directly in front of the participant. Leaning over, the trainer places the palm of each hand on the bar, directly outside the participant's hands. The grip should remain firm but open to allow the bar to roll during the movement. The trainer should then lean over, so that his or her chest is directly above the bar. The trainer's arms remain straight and perpendicular to the floor, creating leverage.

The Movement

The participant begins the movement with the wrists in the down (extended) position, and curls upward as far as possible. During the eccentric phase, the participant slowly returns to the starting position, resisting the trainer. The movement is completed when the participant can no longer curl the wrists upward.

The trainer provides resistance by keeping his or her arms straight and allowing the participant to push the body slightly upward. The trainer maintains leverage by keeping his or her chest above the bar (the rotation axis). Resistance is provided largely by the trainer's body weight.

14.

The Use of Anaerobic-Aerobic Combinations in HRT

The development and refinement of HRT marks a step forward in the fitness and sports field due in large part to the fact that no mechanical equipment is necessary for participation. Aerobic exercise, on the other hand, traditionally has not suffered from the burden of being equipment-specific.

Typically, aerobic exercise is very easy to engage in. It is only in the last thirty years, during the boom in fitness, which spawned the subsequent gyms, fitness centers, and home gyms, that aerobic activity has increasingly included mechanized components. Primarily, this is the result of the need to conserve space — and therefore money. While most aerobic exercise requires little to no equipment, it tends to have at least moderate space requirements. Because of the space/cost issue, most fitness centers are organized in a compact and efficient manner. Similarly, people who choose to work out at home generally do not have the means to build a running track or a basketball court in his or her house.

Equipment Use

The advent of the treadmill, still the most popular piece of equipment in the gym, along with stair steppers, climbers, and elliptical motion machines have allowed for aerobic fitness to occur with minimal space requirements. Additionally, the resulting compact arrangement of aerobic and anaerobic machines allows users to move from one piece of equipment to another quickly, providing a higher quality workout period. While the problem of space has been resolved, the new reliance on mechanization has brought about new problems. The foremost of which is the repetition of a singular action — which most often leads to boredom as the user tries to work through 10-30 minutes aerobic exercise. Although aerobic machines have become increasingly sophisticated, with adjustments that have allowed for changes in speed, elevation, and resistance, they are still only capable of facilitating a singular repetitive motion. The exception being the elliptical motion machine which allows for both forward and backward movement. The end result of increased mechanization is a trade off of space requirements for a lack of variety.

While a decrease in variety leads to a less interesting workout (which can lead to a lack of desire for fitness activities), it is generally acceptable to people who like to combine strength training

Table 14.1. Sample exercise sequence sets

Sample Sequence 1	Sample Sequence 2	Sample Sequence 3
[Jumping Jacks]	[Jump-Ups]	[Mountain Climbers]
Leg Extension	Rows	Push-Ups
Power Squat	Glute Raises	Biceps Curl
Incline Bench	Boxer Crunch	Press-Downs
Hamstring Curls	Bench Press	
Wall Squats	Triceps Press	[Jumping Jacks]
Pull Ups		
Calf Raise	[Rest Period]	Upright Row
Bench Press		Side Raise
Shoulder Press		Resisted Crunch
[Rest Period]		[Rest Period]

and aerobic activities. However, it can be far more detrimental to people who use HRT, which relies on speed, variety, and a lack of equipment. For those interested in periodized training, cross training, and sport specific kinds of workouts, reliance on aerobic machines during training may prove to be somewhat frustrating. After all, who wants to stop in the middle of a workout to boot up a treadmill? It is for this reason that we have included simple, space saving aerobic activities, which don't require equipment and can be inserted at any time during a HRT workout. For these exercises, the trainer's role is greatly decreased, as they perform primarily as a spotter, timing the activity, taking active heart rates, and in general ensuring the safety of the participant.

What are the right times to incorporate aerobic exercises into an HRT workout? There are no set times in which aerobic exercise must be used, if at all. It is entirely up to the trainer's or participant's discretion. They could be done at the start of a routine or set, at the beginning or anywhere in between. For people who are untrained or are just starting to work out again, an anaerobic-aerobic combination may be too stressful for the first few weeks. Table 14.1 on the facing page shows some sample combinations. Aerobic exercises are listed with parentheses. Although the exercises shown in this section are primarily aerobic, most consist of quick ballistic movements in order to rapidly fatigue the participant, providing an anaerobic quality as well. Both the trainer and participant need to be especially careful of previous injuries which could be re-aggravated or could change the form and motion of the exercises, potentially causing a new injury. Pay special attention to the neck, shoulders, lower back, knees, ankles, and feet. Always err on the side of caution and carefully monitor the participant throughout the duration of the exercises.

Knee-Highs

Beginning Position

The participant begins by taking an upright standing position. The feet are shoulder-width apart to provide balance. The chest remains out and the back straight throughout the duration of the exercise.

Movement

At the trainer's signal, the participant performs what is essentially an exaggerated walk in place. Instead of a normal walking motion, the participant brings the knees high, until the top of each leg becomes parallel to the floor at its highest point. If the participant is unable to reach leg height high enough to become parallel to the floor, only go as high as possible without causing discomfort or injury. To increase the difficulty, the participant's arms may be swung upward in an exaggerated motion as well. The exercise should be performed as quickly as possible without losing balance. Knee-highs are typically timed or continued until the desired exercise level is reached.

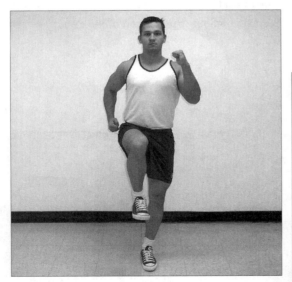

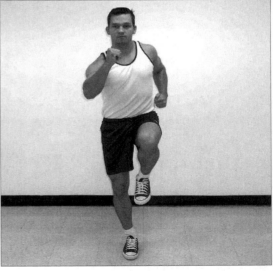

Fig. 14.1. Knee-highs.
Above: starting position.
Right: finishing position.

Mountain Climbers

Beginning Position

The participant should begin by placing his or her hands shoulder-width apart on the floor. This establishes a firm base. Next, it is necessary to move into a "track" stance with the feet shoulder-width apart and offset (one foot in front of the other). The participant should look as if they were at the starting line of a sprint waiting for the signal to begin.

Movement

At the trainer's signal, the participant switches his or her foot positioning in a back and forth motion. Although the participant does not move from the initial beginning position on the floor, the legs move in a back and forth fashion, with each leg moving opposite the other. The exercise should be done as quickly as possible while still maintaining a balanced stance. This can be done as a timed exercise or set to a number of repetitions, either pre-determined or until the desired exercise level is reached.

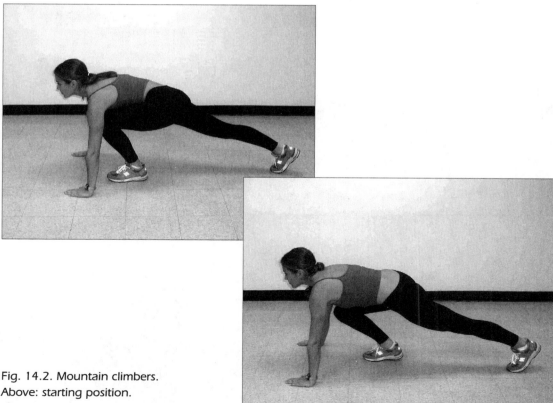

Fig. 14.2. Mountain climbers.
Above: starting position.
Right: finishing position.

Jumping Jacks

Beginning Position

The participant begins the exercise by standing with his or her feet close together and the arms at the sides. The knees should maintain a slightly bent position in order to guard against injury.

Movement

At the trainer's signal, the participant jumps upward, bringing the arms from the sides of the body together over the head. The feet should move outward during the jump, so they are slightly more than shoulder-width apart as the jump is completed. The movement is completed as the participant jumps again, returning to the starting position. Jumping jacks can be done either as a timed exercise or completed upon a certain number of repetitions, with equal effectiveness.

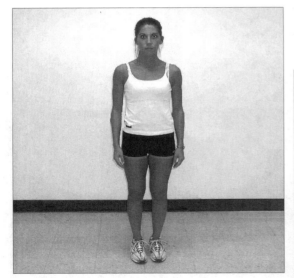

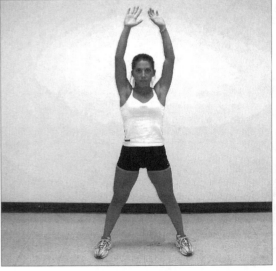

Fig. 14.3. Jumping jacks.
Above: starting position.
Right: finishing position.

Stair Step

Beginning Position

The participant begins by standing in front of a set of stairs or a stable platform. The feet should be shoulder-width apart and within one stride length of the first step.

Movement

At the trainer's signal, the participant should step from the floor onto the first step. After both feet are firmly on the step, the participant steps backward onto the floor with the lead foot first. This action is repeated until the trainer signals the participant to stop. Next, repeat using the opposite leg as the lead leg. This exercise should be done as quickly as possible while maintaining proper balance. The stair step can be done either as a timed exercise or at the trainer's discretion.

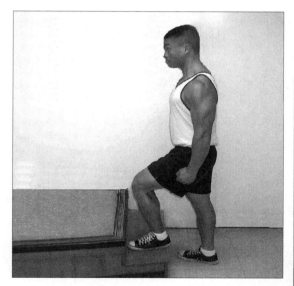

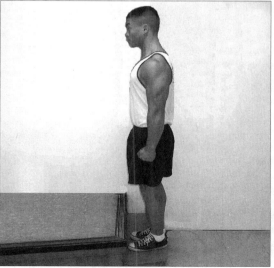

Fig. 14.4. Stair step.
Above: starting position.
Right: finishing position.

Appendix: Fitness Glossary

Abduction — A movement away from the midline (middle) of the body. A side movement such as raising the arm away from the body's center.

Accommodative Resistance — A resistance force that controls the speed of the individual's movement throughout the entire range of motion. Also known as isokinetic resistance, it is the basis of Human Resistance Training

Adaptation — The ability of the body or muscle to adjust to work or resistance.

Adaptation Threshold — The level of adaptation reached when performance fails to increase. The adaptation threshold can only be surpassed by a change in training.

Adduction — A movement toward the midline (middle)of the body. The opposite of abduction.

Aerobic — With or in the presence of oxygen.

Agonistic Muscle — The muscle directly engaged in muscular contraction, primarily responsible for movement.

All-or-Nothing Law — Rule that states when a stimulated nerve fiber contracts, all of the associated muscle fibers contract completely or not at all.

Anabolic — The process of building muscle tissue.

Anaerobic — Without or not requiring the presence of oxygen.

Antagonist Muscle — The muscle that works in direct opposition to the agonistic muscle, by opposing its contraction.

Anterior — The front or toward the front.

Atrophy — The shrinking or decrease in muscle tissue, due to the lack of use or disease.

Axis of Rotation — The imaginary line or point at which an object, such as a lever, rotates.

Ballistic — A dynamic or forceful movement.

Catabolic — The breakdown of body or muscle tissue, where complex substances are reduced to simpler ones.

Central Nervous System (CNS) — The part of the nervous system which consists of the spinal cord and brain

Concentric Contraction — The movement that occurs when the muscle is shortened as a result of contraction during exercise. Also known as the "positive" motion of an exercise.

Connective Tissue — Tissues such as tendons, ligaments, and fascia which bind together forming support for muscle groups.

Delayed Onset Muscle Soreness (DOMS) — The muscle soreness that typically occurs 24 to 48 hours after exercise. Most often associated with eccentric muscle contraction (negative motion)during exercise.

Detraining — The opposite of muscle adaptation. The effects of detraining occur more rapidly than gains made during training (exercise) and are most evident in strength and stamina reduction. Typically occurs two weeks after the last exercise session.

Eccentric Contraction — The movement that occurs when the muscle is lengthened during exercise. Also known as the "negative" motion of an exercise.

Fixators — Muscles that when stimulated, act to stabilize the position of the bone to perform a motion. Also known as stabilizers.

Flexors — Groups of muscles that cause flexion in the limbs, reducing or decreasing the angle of a joint.

Flexibility — The range of motion of a joint and the related muscle groups. Stretching increases the length and flexibility of muscles, reducing the risk of injuries.

Human Resistance Training (HRT) — A training technique in which the resistance during exercise is provided by trainer (also called spotter or helper), often in conjunction with gravity. Although small items such as rod, towels, belts, stairs, etc. may be used, equipment bearing significant weight cannot. Also known as Manual Resistance Training.

Hypertrophy — An increase in the size of muscle tissue due to an increase in cell size (as opposed to cell number). The opposite of atrophy, hypertrophy occurs in response to strength training.

Intensity — The qualitative expression of strength training indicating how hard the body should be working to stress muscle tissue in order to achieve progressive training effects.

Interval Training — A method of training with variable and intermittent work, containing rest periods. changes can be made to intensity, speed, rest and work length in order to simulate certain sports or athletic events. Interval Training can be used with specific emphasis on the aerobic or anaerobic system.

Isokinetic Contraction — Type of contraction where tension and speed are controlled throughout the range of motion even though maximal force is exerted.

Isometric Contraction — Type of contraction in which the muscle develops tension but where no mechanical work is performed. Shortening and lengthening does not occur but the force output is equal to the resistance. Also known as a static contraction.

Isotonic Contraction — Type of contraction where the muscle shortens (a "positive" movement is performed) against a constant load or resistance, resulting in movement.

Joint — The junction point of two or more bones in the body, forming a functional relationship.

Ligament — A strong band of non-elastic connective tissue used to connect bone to bone, often forming the stabilizing portion of a joint.

Macrocycle — A training phase or cycle which has a duration of approximately 2–8 weeks.

Microcycle — A training phase or cycle which has a duration of approximately 1-week.

Microtears — Small microscopic tears found in muscle tissue, ligaments, and tendons, most often caused by strenuous strength training. As a response to microtears, the body adapts by becoming stronger.

Muscular Strength — The maximum amount of force which can be generated by a muscle or muscle group.

Neural Adaptation — The increase in coordination of the nervous system in response to stressors such as exercise. Often, an untrained or detrained exercise participant will experience rapid neural adaptation during the first six to eight weeks of exercise.

One Repetition Maximum (1-RM)	The maximum amount of weight a person can lift one time, through a range of motion, with proper form, before the muscle cannot successfully perform again.	Rest Interval	The period of time between exercises in a program. Rest Intervals are most specific during the use of Interval Training.
Overload	Principle of training which describes the need to increase the workload (resistance) to levels beyond the current threshold but within the limits of safety to cause beneficial muscle adaptations.	Set	A grouping of repetitions (number of times completed) of a specific movement. For example, a set of hamstring curls may consist of 10 repetitions.
Phase-Specific	A phase or segment of training in which a particular aspect is emphasized (muscle power, definition, hypertrophy, etc.).	Specificity	A type of training which emphasizes a muscle adaptation toward a particular skill or activity. For example, strength training with heavy resistance tends to lead toward hypertrophy while endurance training tends to lead toward greater definition.
Physical Activity	Characterizes all types of physical human movement.	Spotter	Another term for "trainer" or "helper": the individual who watches or assists the participant (also called "lifter" or "client") while the exercise is performed. In HRT, the spotter performs in the active rather than the passive capacity during most exercises.
Plateau	A point during training in which no observable gains are made from the current exercise routine or phase.		
Posterior	Back or toward the back.		
Power	The rate of work over a period of time. Expressed as Power = Work / time ($P = W / t$)	Tendon	A dense fiber bundle that connects muscle tissue to bone. Tendons transmit the muscle's force to the bone.
Prime Movers	The muscle or set of muscles which are primarily responsible for the technical movement in an exercise.	Variable Resistance Exercise	An exercise in which the level of resistance varies at different points throughout the movement. This is commonly found in exercise machines, or equipment such as bands or tubes.
Progressive Resistance Exercise (PRE)	A training technique in which muscles must work against increases of a workload (resistance, frequency, repetitions, duration, interval time).	Work	Physical effort expressed as the product of force and the distance which that force moves. Expressed as Work = Force x Distance ($W = F \times D$).
Repetition	The number of times a specific movement is repeated within a single set.		

The Human Resistance Trainers' Association (HRTA)

The HRTA is the only certifying organization for Human Resistance Training.

- Limited class sizes

- Point by point instruction

- Proper HRT techniques for safe, effective use

- Designed for professionals to use in multiple settings

- Taught by the leading HRT experts

For more information, log on to: http://www.in-fit.com

Index